Psyche, Self and Soul

For Julia, Paul, Connie, Eric, and Nicole

Psyche, Self and Soul

Rethinking Psychoanalysis, the Self and Spirituality

by

GERALD J. GARGIULO PH.D.

W
WHURR PUBLISHERS
LONDON AND PHILADELPHIA

© 2004 Whurr Publishers Ltd
First published 2004
by Whurr Publishers Ltd
19b Compton Terrace
London N1 2UN England and
325 Chestnut Street, Philadelphia PA 19106 USA

Reprinted 2005

British Library Cataloguing in Publication Data

A catalogue record for this book
is available from the British Library.

ISBN 10- 1 86156 443 0 p/b
ISBN 13- 978 1 86156 443 6 p/b

Typeset by Adrian McLaughlin, a@microguides.net

Contents

Acknowledgments

This text was many years in the making. How difficult, consequently, to acknowledge all the teachers and colleagues who have helped me with their friendship, knowledge, and support. Of my undergraduate teachers, Fr. Ernest Larkin and the late Fr. Francis Donahue were men of profound depth and genuine caring. Among my postgraduate professors, my admiration for Dr Ewert Cousins of Fordham University is paramount; it is the rare teacher who allows you to know what you know.

There are simply too many of my colleagues and friends in the psychoanalytic community with whom I have shared ideas and life over the past 35 years for me to acknowledge them all by name. I am grateful for the opportunity to have studied with Theodor Reik at the National Psychological Association for Psychoanalysis Training Institute and to have worked at *The Psychoanalytic Review* with Dr Martin Schulman. My affiliation with the International Federation for Psychoanalytic Education over the past 14 years has brought me into contact with many wonderful individuals and given me the opportunity to present some of the chapters I have included in this text.

Erika Duncan, of Sag Harbor, has been helpful over the many years of our friendship in refining my writer's voice. Dr Jon Mills, Dr Jeffrey Rubin, and Mr Laurence Chollet have read different portions of the present text and have been generous with their time and insightful with their suggestions. I am likewise appreciative of the generous response given the manuscript by Dr John Morgan of Foundation House, Oxford.

To Dr James Grotstein, I owe special thanks. His writings have stimulated many of my own thoughts, and his generosity of spirit is a continuous source of encouragement.

Mrs Gaylene Gasparini and Mr Kenneth Schwartz have been more than generous with help when computer problems arose; a special thanks to Martha Ayim for her exceptional editorial and computer expertise.

Any psychoanalyst knows that we are taught not just by our studies but by our patients as well: to those I have been able to help, I feel equally rewarded; to those who have looked past my shortcomings and errors, I am indebted.

My children, Paul and Connie, ground my coming and my going; their joy for life is a gift. Finally, to my wife of 40 years, Julia, I owe a special gratitude. She has been my editor, my best critic, and a constant source of strength, insight, and encouragement, quietly loving and real in all these many tasks.

I want to especially acknowledge the gracious permission of Dr Martin Schulman, editor, to reprint from and/or adapt any of my previously published articles in *The Psychoanalytic Review*. The following chapters have all been reprinted with permission:

- An earlier version of 'Meaning and metaphor in psychoanalysis' appeared in *The Psychoanalytic Review* (Gargiulo, 1998a).
- An earlier version of 'Aloneness in psychoanalysis and spirituality' appeared in *International Journal of Applied Psychoanalytic Studies* (Gargiulo, 2004) and has been adapted for this book.
- 'Authority, the self, and psychoanalytic experience' appeared in *The Psychoanalytic Review* (Gargiulo, 1989).
- 'Language, love, and healing' appeared in *Journal of Religion and Health* (Gargiulo, 1999).
- An earlier version of 'Reflections, musings, and interventions: A personal communication on psychoanalytic work' appeared in *Psychoanalysis Today* (Gargiulo, 1991), and has been adapted for this book.
- An earlier version of 'Recollection, empathy, and reverie' appeared in *Dimensions of Empathic Therapy*, P Breggin, G Breggin, F Bemak (eds) Springer Publishing Company Inc. New York 10012. Adapted with permission.
- 'Anna O: An English object relations approach' is from *Anna O.: Fourteen contemporary reinterpretations* (Gerald J. Gargiulo, 1984, pp. 149–160). © 1984, The Free Press, a division of Simon & Schuster Adult Publishing Group. All rights reserved.
- 'Winnicott's psychoanalytic playground' appeared in *Psychoanalytic Versions of the Human Condition* (Gargiulo, 1998b).

- 'Sublimation: Winnicottian reflections' appeared in *The Psychoanalytic Review* (Gargiulo, 1992). The present chapter has been significantly revised.
- 'A modern dialogue with Freud' appeared in *The Psychoanalytic Review* (Gargiulo, 1971a).
- Appendix B, 'Who is the dreamer who dreams the dream?', appeared in *The Psychoanalytic Review* (Gargiulo, 2001).
- Sections of Chapter 4 are taken from a previous article that appeared in *Soul on the Couch*, The Analytic Press, pp. 1–9 (Gargiulo, 1977). All rights reserved.

Finally I acknowledge the permission granted for use of the following poems in the text:

- Excerpts from 'Burnt Norton' from *Four Quartets* by TS Eliot, © 1936 by Harcourt Inc. and renewed 1964 by TS Eliot, reprinted by permission of the publisher. Copyright by permission of Faber and Faber Ltd.
- Excerpts from 'Little Gidding' from *Four Quartets*, © 1942 by TS Eliot and renewed 1970 by Esme Valerie Eliot, reprinted by permission of Harcourt Inc. Copyright by permission of Faber and Faber Ltd.

About the author

Gerald J. Gargiulo PhD, received his doctorate in Psychoanalysis and Spirituality from Foundation House, Oxford. He is a member of the International Psychoanalytical Association and the American Psychoanalytic Association. He is a former president of the Training Institute of the National Psychological Association for Psychoanalysis, a founding member and former president of the International Federation for Psychoanalytic Education and a Fellow of the Council of Psychoanalytic Psychotherapists. He is a Diplomate of the American Psychotherapy Association, a member of Division 39 (Psychoanalysis) of The American Psychological Association and an associate editor of *The Psychoanalytic Review* and *Contemporary Psychoanalytic Studies*. Dr. Gargiulo has lectured internationally, particularly on the work of D. W. Winnicott, has published over sixty-five articles and reviews in journals and contributed numerous chapters to books. He co-edited *Soul on the Couch* (Analytic Press). Dr. Gargiulo maintains a private practice in Greenwich, Connecticut, and East Hampton, New York.

Foreword

Psychoanalysis is a living entity. It has its own life force or entelechy, its hidden sense of destiny, and its unpredictable trajectory as it relentlessly evolves. Most of the contributions it receives are from its adherents who are unknowingly frozen in the immediacy of their Zeitgeist, unaware that their contributions are dated and obsolescent as soon as they are published because psychoanalysis, as a living entity, has moved on even while they wrote. A great portion of psychoanalytic contributions is *scientific* in nature, but *science* gauges only measurable systems, not non-linear or complex systems. What psychoanalysis needs are those rare pilots who can intuit its *soul* and thereby be able to discern its ever-changing course as it relentlessly evolves. Bion uses the term *mystic* or *genius* to identify such rare individuals who naturally face the Absolute Truth about Ultimate Reality. Bion goes farther: he believes that psychoanalysis is a *mystic science.*

Gargiulo's work is that of psychoanalytic mystic. A mystic is not one who mystifies. He is one who sees clearly through the camouflage of images and symbols that stand between the subject and the object: *Now through a glass darkly; then face to face*. The background that informs his work is quite impressive. Before becoming a trained psychoanalyst he was an associate professor of religious studies and a student, for many years, of Carmelite spirituality. The North Star of his work is Donald Winnicott, who ranks, in my opinion, as one of the three psychoanalytic mystics of the past century, the other two being Bion and Lacan. What is a psychoanalytic mystic? It is one who eschews the known cant of a body of knowledge, *turned dogma* – along with its three-dimensional, linear outlook (i.e., transference, resistance, psychic apparatus, etc.) – for a mystical outlook, one that deals with emptiness, contemplation, infinity, chaos, unpredictability, spirituality, and immanence.

Spirituality and immanence deserve further discussion. Freud and his positivistic legacy offered no room for theology, philosophy, spirituality, or godliness, except as psychopathology. Gargiulo, particularly with his understanding of metaphor, is one of the newer psychoanalysts who seek to rectify that serious omission. Another star on Gargiulo's compass is Meister Eckhart, the thirteenth-century mystic who wrote, 'the eye with which I see God is the same eye with which he sees me'. In my own work, which the author was gracious to cite, I argue that the unconscious is as close to God as any mortal is likely to get. What psychoanalysts have forgotten, but not Gargiulo, is that the unconscious is enshrouded in mystery, can never be known, is ineffable, and is the consummate *subject* – it, like God, who also is the consummate subject, can never be objectified; it can never be known or contemplated. It can only, in Bion's words, be *become*, i.e., experienced.

Let me state this another way. When one trains to become a psychoanalyst, one learns to accept the analysand's free associations, the first reading of which is mysterious, and then places a grid of theory (i.e., the Oedipus complex, castration anxiety, etc.) upon them to give them coherent meaning. The mystical psychoanalyst will not look for those associations that all too comfortably correspond to his or her preconceptions. The mystical psychoanalyst will look solely toward the mystery without preconception, memory, or desire, and allow him- or herself to be immersed in a *cloud of unknowing* until an intuition or an epiphany occurs within, which authentically emerges from an emptiness of mind. To me that is the true psychoanalysis of *this* forthcoming Zeitgeist.

Gargiulo speaks of creativity and of *everyday transcendence*. Following Winnicott, he believes that the analysand, like the infant, must imaginatively *create* the world of objects he or she is in the process of discovering – and that all psychoanalytic theories as well as interpretations constitute ongoing creations – rather than being cemented in fact. Creativity has far-reaching consequences for psychoanalysis. The author enlightens us with the revolutionary – but credible – idea that the unconscious is a creation, not a fact! Everyday transcendence represents the daily experience in ridding oneself of the false idols of imprisoning images, symbols, and preconceptions so as to allow one to be generatively free and able to achieve an at-one-ment with the other and to be able to contemplate a world of infinite possibilities.

In ancient Greece, philosophers did not just *teach* philosophy; they *lived* it. I feel that this is the idea that the author is promulgating in this extraordinary work. He is urging us psychoanalysts to live and practice according to a more enlightened mode of tolerance, a tolerance of not knowing while truth ultimately finds us. He states: 'as therapists we are not only midwives of memory and meaning, but we are . . . midwives of hope and possibility.'

The author has written a beautiful, elegant, and profound work that gets to the soul of psychoanalysis, an aspect of psychoanalysis that is too seldom addressed. It informs psychoanalytic theory and technique in a way that is rare but most welcome. The time for the author's ideas to be appreciated has arrived.

James Grotstein, MD

Preface

Psychoanalysis has shown that the most intellectual academic pursuits have their roots in personal history and that theories are as much related to insight as to personal experience. Psychoanalysis has also taught us that one need not hide life's injuries – they are our common lot. One of Freud's most basic convictions was that there is universality to individuality; given that insight, he could write his *The Interpretation of Dreams*. My own reflections about my personal history, about how and why we relate to each other and the world, about why we tell stories to each other as we seek a truth that finds us, just as we find it, are as personal, in a sense, as my dreams, yet as universal as the human condition. While confessional exhibitionism is unproductive, personal history can help locate the roots and/or inspiration of a person's actions. With this in mind, I would like to highlight some of my life experiences that have propelled me to explore not only psychoanalysis but also spirituality.

I had a strong-willed, hard working, but difficult father. While I admired his work ethic, I found his incapacity to relate, with any sense of personal vulnerability, frustrating. My early years, consequently, were marked by a low-grade depression that manifested itself in difficulties with learning, complicated by frequent physical illnesses. During my adolescence, a midlife crisis in my mother's life further complicated my own depression. I knew I was looking for an ideal by which I could mold and define my life. By age 18, one year into college, I decided to enter a Roman Catholic monastic order to pursue studies for the priesthood. This life choice, which lasted 10 years, included disciplined study, respectful peer companionship, and sensible and caring teachers, all of which were reparative for my sense of self. But it did not ultimately ground that self. Sensing that I should pursue a different life path, I decided, with the therapeutic help of a sensitive psychiatrist, to leave the monastery immediately priory to any ordination to the priesthood. I became a lay professor of religious studies at a northeastern college. During my eight years as a college professor, I married, started a family, undertook doctorate courses at Fordham University and completed my studies at a psychoanalytic training institute founded by Theodor Reik, and opened a private practice. (A more detailed summary will be found in my essay 'Remembering a Quiet Place' in *Why I became a Psychotherapist* (Gargiulo, 1998c).)

Years of clinical practice and teaching at various psychoanalytic institutes followed, complemented by the many administrative roles I held in these organizations. Although my professional life was very rewarding, I came to realize that psychoanalysis and psychoanalysts, not unlike religion and its adherents, were also tempted to offer inherited formulas and dogmatic solutions. Chapter 6, which opens Section 2, 'Clinical studies: in search of a self', reflects my response to such approaches and outlines the ground place out of which I believe any therapy must flow. Chapters 7 and 8 evidence my working through some of the mechanistic approaches I had been taught in the process of coming to know how two people listen to each other and heal their wounds. In this vein, Chapter 9 is a retrospective – looking back at Anna O. 100 years later. Each of the three sections of the text, although related in theme, can be read separately.

The works of Donald Winnicott became crucial in my progressive understanding and practicing. Section 3 of this book, 'D.W. Winnicott', focuses on his work; Chapter 10, 'Winnicott's psychoanalytic playground', outlines his major contributions and Chapter 11, 'Sublimation: Winnicottian reflections', shows his understanding of play and its relationship to the traditional psychoanalytic concept of sublimation. Rather than finding the truth, a *Weltanschauung* that answers life's riddles, I have attempted to share my experience of several truths, which one can experience as normative without being coercive. Winnicott's reliance on paradox helps clarify such an approach. In this vein I speak about a sense of one's own internality, that alone place within us, as the prerequisite for knowing the world. In therapy, the search within ideally ushers in a deeper contact with the world. It is within such a framework that I offer an understanding of the relationship between psychoanalysis and spirituality; they are both disciplines that attempt to explore internality. I discuss this relationship in Chapters 1–5, in Section 1. An individual's sensitivity to and awareness of his or her internality is the best safeguard against neurotic repetition, as well as the best grounding for a spirituality that is rooted in Mother Earth and not the heavens above. The experience of internality, as is obvious, is equally applicable to a therapist as it is to a patient; the result of therapy, as I discuss in Chapter 5, should issue in a true egalitarian experience, i.e., the resolution of transference and countertransference means a sober acknowledgment of the respective benefits and mishaps that both patient and analyst have brought to their encounter. Anything less is the perpetuation of a religious, in contrast to a spiritual, experience.

Historically psychoanalytic writers have been suspicious of any positivistic religious statements and/or of a spirituality that focuses on visions or heavenly revelations, any of which promise personal specialness. Rightly so. But to exclusively focus on such phenomena is to miss a significant aspect of human reality. When Winnicott, toward the end of his life, wrote, 'O God, when I die, may I be alive' (C. Winnicott, 1989, p. 4), he was not praying, I believe, to any absolute transcendent Other who created and rules the world. Only when we can sense the depth that is within us, an openness that transcends the repressed unconscious, will we be able to experience the depth that surrounds us. I introduce the concept of an 'everyday transcendence' – a reality that is within our world yet outside our immediate experience, a primordial backdrop, as it were, to our actions, as an approach to understanding what I mean by 'depth'. In order to find an apt metaphor for an everyday transcendence, I have employed, as a layman in theoretical physics, the quantum-mechanics notion of a *mist of infinite possibilities*.[1] The world that we experience is constantly coming to be, as we are constantly coming to be, and we all have a hand in this ongoing creation. I find the concept of a mist of infinite possibilities a sober antidote to our tendency to reify our theories or beliefs.

---

1 Note Greene's (2000, p. 420) definition of quantum mechanics as a 'framework of laws governing the universe whose unfamiliar features such as *uncertainty, quantum fluctuations*, and *wave-particle duality* become most apparent on the microscopic scales of *atoms* and subnuclear particles'. And Gregory (1988, p. 98), on a more popular level, notes, 'Quantum mechanics is a way of talking about nature that allows physicists to predict how the world will respond to being measured'. Niels Bohr noted: 'There is no quantum world. There is only an abstract quantum physical description . . . Physics concerns only what we can *say* about nature' (as quoted in Gregory, 1988, p. 95). A *mist of infinite possibilities* is a way of talking about a world of probabilities, a world that is a backdrop, a ground to what we experience, a world that I speak of, particularly in Chapter 2, as a vital emptiness.

I inform my discussion of the unconscious by this perspective of infinite possibilities. I see what we name as the unconscious as a bridge leading both nowhere and everywhere. Such indeterminateness is not a seedbed for a cynical relativism; an experience of creativity, individual and collective, is a more desirable and engaging alternative.

Throughout Chapters 2–4, I play, in Winnicott's sense, with the concept of 'the unconscious' and the notion of a personal 'I' as well as offer an alternative perspective on the concept of 'mind'. I am not the first to note the profound misconceptions of reality that abound whenever one does not understand psychoanalytic or spiritual concepts metaphorically; I present, particularly in these chapters, alternative metaphors for an understanding of such concepts. Knowledge, I believe, is a communal experience, not a private commodity; I offer such reflections as an invitation to further speculation.

The particular tradition of spirituality that I refer to is known as the *negative*, or *apophatic, way* – a tradition of spirituality that has its roots, in the west, in Neoplatonism. This tradition emphasizes human unknowingness and the need to recognize and to stay within such unknowingness. I refer frequently to Meister Eckhart, the thirteenth-century mystic, philosopher, and theologian, as my primary source for this tradition. Unknowingness is something psychoanalysts, in particular, should be at home with. Appendix A is a study of Paul Ricoeur's *Freud and Philosophy*, which locates Freud's contributions within the context of western thought while also giving a hermeneutical reading to his writings. As I note in my review, 'to say that humans are incomplete is to comment on our historicity; to notice defects is to appreciate evolution, and to speak of evil is to be aware that power, in its many forms, may go astray' – by which I mean to focus on a spirituality that is grounded in the here and now and a psychoanalysis that acknowledges history and thereby its own limitations. Appendix B offers a detailed review of Dr James Grotstein's *Who Is the Dreamer Who Dreams the Dream?* My encounter with his text was an invitation to explore many of the observations I develop in Section 1.

To create the found world, which as Winnicott suggests is a perennial human task, is to understand that culture is more a playground for humanity's dreams than a jailer of its desires. It is to know that we must love the world, if it is going to be real for us; that we only find our own voice as we are able to hear another's. I have attempted in this text to let psychoanalysis hear other voices – be that the voice of

Eckhart or the reflections/speculations of quantum mechanics. Psychoanalysis has taught us that only when we can freely hear can we know who we are.

Gerald J. Gargiulo
March 2004

SECTION 1
THEORETICAL REFLECTIONS

CHAPTER 1

Meaning and metaphor in psychoanalysis[1]

The minute we begin to talk about this world, however, it somehow becomes transformed into another world, an interpreted world, a world delimited by language.

Bruce Gregory (1988, p. 183)

It is more than an academic question if we ask, in the tradition of Theodor Reik, whether we can train someone to be a psychoanalyst or whether psychoanalysts are, in fact, born. Since we generally act as if we can train an individual to competently, and even occasionally to creatively, practice this art form, I would like to focus on the latter alternative, namely, psychoanalysts are born. (This position might endanger the financial viability of most psychoanalytic training institutes, but for the present I leave such a consideration aside.) If we speak of analysts as born to be such, I am not implying some divine election or mystery cult priesthood. What I am wondering about is the implication for our field if we say that the capacity to practice analysis precedes any formal training, as such, and is actually a prerequisite for effectively and creatively using the training at all. By training I include personal analysis, which, although vital for any psychoanalyst to experience, is nevertheless subordinate to certain individual qualities: primarily a capacity for personal honesty, a desire for cross-identification issuing in compassion and civility, and the possession of what we may call a playful intelligence. Unfortunately we have no way of guaranteeing the acquisition of these qualities, despite the length of any analysis.

The quality that I would like to emphasize is the need to possess a playful intelligence; I mention the other qualities, however, as a

---

1 This is a revised version of the 1997 Presidential Address at the IFPE Conference at Ann Arbour, MI.

context for understanding my reflections. Much of psychoanalytic education has undervalued the need for these overall character traits as prerequisites for practicing psychoanalysis, emphasizing instead content mastery and/or the completion of clinical/therapeutic requirements. To pursue that line of thought, however, would require a separate chapter.

I introduce my thoughts about metaphor and meaning in psychoanalytic education by recounting a personal experience. Many years ago a colleague and I, both new to the field, were participating in a public discussion with a psychologist, a professor of phenomenological psychology, who was presenting his clinical work. At one point, my colleague asked the speaker, rather pointedly, whether or not he believed in the unconscious. This was done, I suspect, to ascertain how psychoanalytically informed the presenter was. Although I thought I understood the thrust of the question, I was troubled by its turn of phrase. I had, a few years prior, left many years of studying and teaching theology. I wondered, on hearing my colleague's question, whether I had stumbled somehow back onto an old route, a route where the personal acknowledgment of belief in the unconscious, or the oedipal complex, for example, ultimately determined one's affiliation or, more ominously, one's correctness. Such an approach is comparable to asking whether one believes that one's religious scriptures are a product of divine revelation.

Over my years as a teacher and student of psychoanalysis, I have heard, in various garbs, the same kind of formulation. Not infrequently I would hear colleagues talk about the acceptance of the oedipal complex as the core of neurosis, as a defining prerequisite for practicing psychoanalysis. Another shibboleth by which to prove whether one is a true psychoanalyst is the acknowledgment of a particular formulation for the concept of transference. I do not wish to beg the question by isolating certain religiously toned words and to question their usage. The problem is more troubling. I understand the personal yearning we all share for a body of knowledge, for something to know with certainty. Although such knowledge has some functional usefulness, it is, in fact, both intellectually and existentially dangerous – dangerous, because psychoanalysis is primarily a metaphor, perhaps a key metaphor, for understanding many of the other metaphors that comprise our intellectual, cultural, and personal lives.

Although we speak of psychoanalysis as a theory of the mind – a mode of investigation as well as a clinical technique – without understanding it as a metaphor, we are in danger of knowing a great deal while understanding very little. Any theory, or model of the mind, separated from its grounding as a living 'metaphor' is, in effect, an Eden-laden apple, more seductive than the rise and fall of our libidinal fantasies.

By metaphor I do not mean exclusively a figure of speech but rather a primary route to the experience of meaning. The metaphors of psychoanalysis, in either their traditional Freudian formulations or the other various alternative or complementary formulations, can be experienced as discoveries, i.e., Freud discovered the unconscious or transference, or as creative formulations meant to evoke and suggest an interesting way of organizing human experience. I do not believe that one discovers the unconscious or transference comparable to discovering the bones of *Homo habilis* in the layered mud of Africa, or a purposefully hidden treasure. It is more useful to speak of the unconscious and transference, for example, as phenomena that are experienced as they are interpreted. They are created by interpretation. Even our understanding of the dynamic unconscious, with its notion of force/counterforce and the return of the repressed, is, obviously, not comparable to the forces/counterforces in a gas-driven engine. It is a metaphor, among many, indicating our paradoxical capacity to know and not know, to be aware and to turn away from awareness, the latter being the road to illusion.

It is a truism to note that artists and poets not infrequently create the unconscious more effectively than we analysts, particularly to the extent that psychoanalytic education does not encourage playfulness with language and with theory. That western consciousness, for a major portion of the twentieth century, was resonant with Freud's metaphors is well known. His metaphors have been profoundly useful for human reflection; it is hoped that they can continue to be so, only, however, if we understand that what Freud gave form to is what we have to give form to, i.e., if we are not constantly recreating psychoanalysis, we are, in fact, killing it.

What does recreating it mean? Minimally we can say that, unless we are constantly re-finding the metaphorical aspect of our knowledge, we can, all too easily, slip into a literal, concrete understanding of it. If any theoretical formula or model does not impel us to wonder, reflection becomes a dead formula. If we speak of transference, for example, it is important to recognize that knowledge is always provisional, just outside our reach, a little beyond our grasp. Such awareness can help keep our reading of the situation between patient and analyst modest. Minimally we should keep in mind that there are many selves that we all bring to the moment. When we speak of transference, therefore, we are isolating in order to appreciate complexity. Great literature shows us that it is only in the poetic or fictional re-creation of reality that we even get close to it. No wonder Freud said that Dostoevsky was a better psychologist than he! Transference is one such metaphor for our capacity of re-creation; it is pathological when a particular mode of expression overshadows the whole of our many selves, our many varied relationships. To the extent that we do not recognize a metaphorical reading of transference, to the extent that we do not teach it, we are destined, I believe, to fall into what Alfred North Whitehead (1960) calls the error of misplaced concreteness, i.e., mistaking an object as an ultimate reality rather than as a point of reference, attempting to understand a particular event separate from the whole context of its occurrence.

A metaphor is, as we know, that which evokes something else, a use of analogy to promote a depth of meaning and emotional resonance, as when we speak, for example, of the evening of life. Just as a metaphor points to something else, locates the center of meaning somewhere else, we must remember that ultimately there is not, nor can there be, one definitive center of meaning. By the very nature of our capacity to use metaphor, we are guaranteed continuous new meanings. Rather than ask whether a person believes in the unconscious, for example, we would, today, be more interested in what enables a person to believe in anything. To identify something as unconscious, for example, is to attempt to contextualize an individual's self-understanding. When we say that the unconscious is revealed or found *as it is interpreted*, we are describing an aspect of self-knowledge that comes in many guises. Knowing oneself is also to experience not knowing oneself, turning our eyes away from, or even refusing to see, oneself.

How can we speak of such paradoxical knowing? We can effectively use the model of the unconscious as long as we recognize and help our students to recognize that we are neither accepting a psychoanalytic dogma nor postulating a *deus ex machina*. In this sense the unconscious is always a metaphor for the inevitably hidden in human discourse and experience, for the hidden that we both actively perpetuate and are arbitrarily subject to.

The metaphorical nature of the unconscious is equally true of such concepts as resistance, transference, idealized self-object, or transitional space. We can also speak, in a Lacanian framework, of desire itself as a metaphor for the other, i.e., the other as culture, the other that germinates desire within us; even the prohibition of desire is the other as superego. If we forget such considerations and proceed as if we can analyze desire as a singular possession, we are in danger, as analysts, of mishearing. In this vein I am reminded of what Italo Calvino (1974) wrote in his masterful *Invisible Cities*, namely, 'it is not the voice that commands the story: it is the ear' (p. 106). We need poets, midwives of metaphor, to help us hear what a patient is saying.

Further, if we proceed as if we can analyze desire as singular, we are also in danger, as Winnicott (1958) has written, of confusing mind and psyche. As I (Gargiulo, 1997) have written elsewhere, when we speak of mind we can avoid limiting our understanding by not reducing it to brain, or imagination, or memory, or to thinking in terms of problem-solving. As I use the term, 'mind' is more than singular, more than an individual's personal possession. Without understanding its communal base, as particularly but not exclusively exemplified in our use of language, without appreciating how we are given a sense of *I-ness* by the particular culture we live in, we can easily over-premise individuality and be blind to what mind, in all its metaphorical referents, can stand for.

In a different context, Otto Fenichel, a master of Freudian theory, was acutely aware of the danger of analyzing the singular, of concretizing the individual, when he wrote:

Neuroses are the outcome of unfavorable and socially determined educational measures, corresponding to a given and historically developed social milieu and necessary in this milieu. They cannot be changed without corresponding change in the milieu.

Fenichel (1945, p. 586)

Are we doing a service to the truth, and to our students, if we teach about defenses, about transference, about being alive, and talk as if we are describing phenomena solely locatable within individuals and expressed simply by that individual's personal history? If we can speak about the 'I' as a cultural/imaginative construct, is not the 'I' then a metaphor for that culture and all the forces – intellectual, economic, artistic, religious, and philosophical – that constitute that culture? Just as the transitional space between mother and child is the ground source for civilization and culture, so the transitional space between analyst and patient should not be reduced to a figurative place inhabited by forgotten teddy bears, or a haven for solipsistic phantasies. It is the ground bed out of which analysts and patients locate their ever-changing center, a center that is a ground space for meaning.

Meaning, as Erik Erikson (1963) has observed, is relative to our life experiences, a point he noted when describing the achievement of human wisdom as manifested in one's capacity to pass on life knowledge while simultaneously recognizing its actual historical relativity. Such a position goes a long way toward modifying our narcissistic need, both as teachers and as students, to know, to have found the way – the Gnostic promise to be counted among the enlightened.

Ultimately, then, it makes no sense to believe in anything if that means forgetting the metaphorical nature of knowledge. Sir Peter Medawar (1982), the English research biologist and philosopher, is not alone when he reminds us that even in the empirical sciences 'a hypothesis is an imaginative preconception of what might be true' (p. 122). In this vein we can no more believe in psychoanalysis than we can believe in cybernetics. I do not mean that as a pejorative comparison. The only way we can practice psychoanalysis is, paradoxically, to recognize the need for a guided praxis while at the same time acknowledging the primacy of perspective over content. That Winnicott or Kohut, for example, have offered alternative perspectives, alternative metaphors, does not negate Freud's perspective. We simply have alternative ways of approaching what we choose to call content, e.g., oedipal desires. Each new perspective is ultimately an act of creation, revealing more by placing what we are addressing in a wider context. Winnicott's (1958) famous dictum that 'there is no such thing as a baby' (p. 99) grounds oedipal desires, for example, more forcefully than any 5-year-old's phantasies. Understanding the metaphorical basis of knowledge frees us of the Herculean burden of finding the truth. We can, instead, settle for a truth or, should I say, several truths. Most of what I read about today, from those who feel that they must kill Freud off, is their belated discovery that he did not possess the truth. Unfortunately, in the history of psychoanalysis other Ur analysts have walked this path. When Winnicott chided Melanie Klein for her insistence that those who recognized her contributions should use only her language, he was arguing for the use of personal metaphors over collective allegiance, for a commitment to a humanistic science rather than a conversion to a new religion.

When we understand transference as a metaphor, as I have mentioned, we are attempting to elucidate how we are contextual creations, made up of our many histories and our many desires. We can appreciate that when patients are, for the psychological moment, their forgotten childhood dreams, fears, hopes, or expectations, they nevertheless encompass more than meets the ear, at that moment. Transference, in this context, is a metaphor for memory, for our need to speak the language spoken to us, for the ambiguity of desire, and sometimes the absence of desire, as well as the different selves desires evoke. That we are formed by our history, and by what we do with that history, is not intrinsically a statement of pathology but of the dilemma of self-understanding. A transference neurosis, consequently, with its narrowing focus on who the analyst is, or is to be, comes about, I believe, precisely because the patient has lost the capacity to know the analyst as metaphor for what the patient needs. The patient collapses into the literal and thereby eclipses the metaphorical.

Finally, in the context of understanding psychoanalytic concepts metaphorically, I would like briefly to comment on the concept of regression. Thinking linearly promotes the image of regression as a back-and-forward phenomenon, as if measuring ego functions on a ruler. Thinking metaphorically allows us to know that there is always another reading, always another affective memory that we can experience; all of which helps us appreciate that personal integration is not simply a landmark developmental achievement so much as an operative goal with constantly varying manifestations. Consequently, how we conceptualize the notion of regression will either tie us to concrete thinking or enable us to grasp the complex simultaneity of human functioning. It is a truism that we live on many levels at once. The concept of regression can be productively understood as an ongoing attempt to capture the obvious complexity of our human functioning, paradoxically, by narrowing our focus.

Now, if we come back to our question of education for psychoanalysts and its possibility, we can again try to understand Reik's thought that psychoanalysts are born and not made. Another way of saying this might be to state that one must, in some way, be a psychoanalyst before starting any formal training if one is to benefit from such training. I believe Freud was thinking in this vein in *The Question of Lay Analysis* when he wrote that analysts should have a 'kind of sharpness for hearing for what is unconscious and repressed, which is not possessed equally by everyone' (Freud, 1926, p. 219). He went on, as we know, to recommend that individuals with a background in history, literature, or the psychology of religion undertake the study and practice of this new science.

By intellectual discipline and/or life experiences, one must be able to transcend the immediacy of the present, the immediacy of the concrete. To be able to appreciate the intrinsic arbitrary selectivity of awareness that any language or cultural modes provide is to experience our symbolizing capacity and to set oneself free from the illusion of certainty. To love the world and to experience personal competence, to value oneself and to be committed to the surprise, again following Reik's lead, of finding out who we are with honesty and humor – these are the qualities needed for the study of psychoanalysis. To study whatever insights a psychoanalytic perspective can provide, knowing, without depression, narcissistic injury, or intellectual cynicism, that we are not able to hold truth except as a point of reference – such are the qualities we need if we are to find ourselves as psychoanalysts.[2]

Winnicott had such issues in mind when he wrote that our first task as analysts is fostering a patient's capacity for play. If we do so, if we encourage the play of metaphor, in all its ramifications with the self, the other, and the world, we will have done more than we can possibly know. To use an old religious and philosophical metaphor, we will have freed the soul from the body, i.e., we will have made life possible, free from living in a world of the concrete, the concreteness of things, the concreteness of thought.

Psychoanalysts are not only midwives of memory but also harbingers of a new future. We can experience our profession as playfully expansive rather than tediously repetitious, as we understand that we live in a sea of meanings, as we understand that we live with a multitude of metaphors.

---

2 Note Freud's (1926) observation, in the Socratic tradition: 'only a man who really knows is modest, for he knows how insufficient his knowledge is' (p. 232).

CHAPTER 2

Aloneness in psychoanalysis and spirituality

We are all part of one another, and we are each just the totality of things seen from our own viewpoint.

Julian Barbour (1999, p. 329)

There is no quantum world, there is only an abstract quantum description.

Niels Bohr (in Wallace, 1996, p. 55)

'Religion', Alfred North Whitehead (1960) wrote, 'is what the individual does with his own solitariness' (p. 16). In this passage, Whitehead gives a particularly profound reading of religion, i.e., he is not speaking of organized belief or ritual practices but of what many today would describe as spirituality. Accepting Whitehead's reflections we can speak of *spirituality* as that area of human experience interested in *exploring individual solitariness.* Such an approach has the benefit of focusing on each individual's task to find what is most real and, consequently, true for him or her. Furthermore, if Donald Winnicott (1958) is right when he speaks of religion and culture, psychoanalysis and play as having their seedbeds in what he categorizes as the *transitional space of childhood*, a transitional space that arises from the experience of *the me and not me* (which postulates, thereby, the essential aloneness of each person), then it is obvious that psychoanalysis is also concerned with the *solitariness of the individual.* How to understand such solitariness is the primary focus of this chapter. My understanding is that both psychoanalysis and spirituality are grounded in such solitariness, in such individual aloneness – an aloneness, a solitariness that is not an isolating and/or disconnecting experience but rather molds, as it were, how one interacts with others as well as with oneself.

Winnicott (1965) writes of a quiet, alone space that each individual possesses and which no one, particularly a psychoanalyst, should attempt to invade.[1] His thoughts on the capacity to be alone, albeit in the presence of the other, reflect not just a developmental achievement but also an existential necessity. Such a capacity to be alone is, as we know, basic to feeling alive and consequently to being able to experience the world as emotionally significant. When Winnicott writes, for example, that many analyses go on for years, under the false assumption that a patient is alive, he was speaking of an individual's capacity to split off emotional contact from such an internal, alone space. Most psychoanalysts, however, have been content to accept Winnicott's notion of such an *alone space* without exploring its implications. Yet that alone space has to be visited, I believe, in order to grasp any meaningful relationship between spirituality and psychoanalysis.

To be internally alone is obviously quite different from being lonely; actually the failure to be internally alone augments loneliness. Nevertheless, it is difficult, given psychoanalytic categories, to grasp the full meaning of what *alone* means. Employing, admittedly poetic, metaphorical imagery, we can begin to approach a definition by saying *that there is a great emptiness within us that is, paradoxically, brimming with life, with vitality, not deadness*. Such a definition goes beyond the common understanding of aloneness, even in Winnicott's sense. It is an aloneness that is open-ended, so to speak, an aloneness that comes closer to what I mean, and what I believe Whitehead means, by solitariness. Such solitariness provides the foundation for being open to both oneself and the world; it is, I would maintain, the bedrock of therapeutic psychoanalytic practice although, obviously, of a different clinical understanding than the resolution of conflict and/or coming to terms with what fate has dealt us. Following many spiritual traditions, such solitariness has been described as a *vital emptiness* rather than a *blank nothingness*. Both eastern spiritual philosophies and western Judeo-Christian philosophers and mystics speak about such a vital emptiness, which is, in their understanding, the foundation or the ground of our being. I explore what such a paradoxical concept as a vital emptiness, which is the wellspring of our solitariness, means, particularly as manifested in such a profound thinker as the thirteenth-century theologian, philosopher, and mystic Meister Eckhart.

---

1 'Each individual is an isolate, permanently non-communicating, permanently unknown, in fact unfound'. Winnicott (1965, p. 187)

The metaphorical or theoretical model one employs ultimately determines whether one characterizes human beings as open or closed systems, so to speak. One can either conceptualize mind and culture as simply an epiphenomenon of brain/body, or one can postulate that *information*, for lack of a better word, underlies all that we experience. Put another way, we can say that mind organizes meaning, and, equally important, that individuality is anchored in an open-ended commonality. Consequently we can say that to know the world is to know what human beings are; alternatively, to know our interiority is to know the world, i.e., we humans are not just living on the Earth – we are, in some sense, the Earth, in its consciousness.

Employing such an open-ended model, we can ask whether such solitary aloneness is, in fact, a variant of the phenomenological description of consciousness. What I have in mind is Sartre's reading of consciousness as emptiness, a consciousness that has no contents but is rather 'a great wind blowing toward objects' (Sartre, 1937, p. 22). Although this is an appealing analog for what I speak of as our solitary interior vital emptiness, what I am attempting to describe is different from the emptiness of 'reflecting consciousness' (Sartre, 1937, p. 44) and more difficult to describe.

Both psychoanalytic and spiritual traditions assume and presumably foster human dignity; each tradition holds to the importance of or, in spiritual language, the sacredness of each person. But what is this based on? Democratic ideals? Or is there a dim perception in our self-awareness that each of us embodies what we can characterize as a personal transcendence. James Grotstein (2000) alludes to what I would like to characterize as an *everyday transcendence* – a transcendence that is not based on religious faith. One approach to understanding such an everyday or natural transcendence is to say that it reflects what I have spoken of as the ground of personal individuality – an individuality that is formed by a *vital open-ended emptiness*. Such a vital open-ended emptiness is, I believe, the basis not only for our solitariness but also for our awareness of personal individual dignity.[2]

To grasp this common or everyday transcendence, I propose a definition that is paradoxical. As our discussion progresses, the need for paradox, in order to appreciate such an everyday transcendence, should be clearer and perhaps less provocative in its formulation. So, then,

---

2 Although many psychoanalysts do not speak in a language that they consider tainted by mysticism, there are a growing number of contemporary analysts, in addition to Grotstein, who are willing to plumb insights coming from spiritual traditions.

we can say that *what is non-existent is truly transcendent*, i.e., a *non-existence* that is alive with what we can further characterize as *unlimited possibilities*. Such a transcendence grounds existence, while not being limited by it. Such a definition echoes Zen Buddhist thought as well as, interestingly, the language of quantum mechanics.[3] For our purposes, and following the language of quantum mechanics, we can speak of *a mist of unlimited possibilities*, which pervades and supports the total reality we humans experience.[4] I am aware that to speak of an alive emptiness of unlimited possibilities that somehow grounds our existence is a particularly difficult, verging on an obtuse, concept. Nevertheless, I think its applicability for understanding the two roads of psychoanalysis and spirituality cannot be minimized. Rather than focusing on the apparent reality or concreteness of the world as a simple given, the postulates of quantum mechanics suggest that the world we experience is a product of our observations, of our questioning. Albert Einstein said as much when he noted, 'It is the theory that decides what we can observe' (in Gregory, 1988, p. 199), a statement that many psychoanalytic practitioners can likewise confirm.

The potential unlimitedness of what we call *reality* is known only piecemeal through our tested observations and the particular line of questioning that informs those observations. I would like to relate what we have spoken of as the vital emptiness (or nothingness) of individual solitariness to the quantum mechanics postulate of an

---

3 Western philosophical tradition has concluded, since the days of Aristotle, that from nothing, nothing comes; eastern Zen Buddhist thought focuses, paradoxically, on the conviction that it is nothingness (the void) that grounds all that is. It has not been until the twentieth century that western theoretical physics has appreciated emptiness or nothingness. Stephen Hawking (1988) speaks of the entire cosmos as possibly coming forth from a vacuum. If the vacuum of the Big Bang turns out to be an unending cycle of expansion and contraction, then the mist of unlimited possibilities (probabilities), which occupies no space or time, will still ground both the void and the ever renewing cosmos. Eastern and Western thought are ultimately angles of vision.

4 For a popular discussion of these concepts, see Kenneth Chang (2000). A theoretical discussion of quantum theory is well developed in Greene (2000). Note, in particular, 'John Wheeler coined the term "quantum foam" to describe the frenzy revealed by such an ultramicroscopic examination of space (and time)' (Greene, 2000, pp. 128–129). Werner Heisenberg initially addressed this issue by noting that 'in every act of perception we select one of the infinite number of possibilities and thus we also limit the number of possibilities for the future.' (as quoted in Beller, 1999, p. 67). Richard Fenyman has termed the phrase 'sum over Histories' (see Hawking, 1988, p. 134 et seq.) to indicate that a proton takes every possible course. Using this concept analogously, we can say that within the *mist of possibilities* the highest probability fosters occurrence. Fenyman, both seriously and humorously, warns the reader against trying to *understand* quantum mechanics, i.e., in this case, how a proton takes every course, even backward in time. For a more popular discussion of Fenyman's ideas see Zukav (1979, p. 230 et seq.).

unlimited mist of possibilities. Such nothingness, such emptiness, is not only the everyday transcendence we are speaking of, but, more to the point, it is the foreground of what we have called the mist of unlimited possibilities. Each individual is an example of, as well as a circumference to, such a mist of unlimited possibilities. What we experience as choice, what we name as *freed-will*, using Edward Glover's (1963) interesting phrase, can be understood as actualizing particular possibilities.[5] This comes about in both psychoanalytic treatment and spiritual journeys through what we can speak of as *a particular history of questioning*. I return to this perspective shortly, but first I want to reiterate that the *emptiness* we are discussing is not barren; nor is the *nothingness* sterile. The emptiness and nothingness that I am speaking of as supporting individual solitariness are an emptiness, a nothingness that can be described as a *natural* or *everyday transcendence* – a natural or everyday transcendence founded, it bears repeating, on the ubiquity of a mist of unlimited possibilities.

It is important to differentiate what Freud (1927) in *The Future of an Illusion* speaks of as an oceanic feeling, a feeling of an undifferentiated merger with the early mother, from what we are classifying as a metaphorical concept, intended to be used as a bridge between our profound interiority and what we experience as our exteriority. To repeat, the solitariness of the individual, which we have in mind, is best captured by the concept of a natural transcendence; if we try to describe this natural transcendence, we are forced back to speaking in terms of nothingness, of emptiness – a potentiality, a void, which each individual concretizes, but which is dense with possibilities.

Both psychoanalysis and spirituality are created and experienced, as disciplines, through their respective and particular history of questioning. Such a history of questioning is how each discipline attempts to reach, react, and respond to individual solitariness. Language, Wittgenstein asserts, forms our world. Gregory (1988), a scientist and writer on astrophysics, notes, 'We might even say the language that we "are" shapes the world, for language undoubtedly defines us more profoundly than we can begin to imagine' (p. 200). In psychoanalysis, even when an analyst is most silent, most neutral, in the

---

5 Glover (1963, p. 193) notes, 'The psychic determinism of Freud at least permits man to hope that in the unending struggles between Id impulse and Ego-adaptation, the victories gained during early development may stand him in good stead. Even if the amount of "freed-will" accruing therefrom is only marginal, it at any rate allows man the freedom to decide to continue the struggle'.

traditional manner, we are helping the patient to learn the language of self and other; both analyst and patient are forging new meanings and consequently finding and relating to a new world. We can reduce psychoanalysis to symptom resolution or to coming to terms with one's history, or, without denying any therapeutic goals, can see it as a new model for understanding the profundity and complexity of human existence. Freud was loath to see his new science as a child of philosophy, but in fact *psychoanalytic man*, in his goals of self-understanding, self-transcendence, and capacity to interact with the world, is a product, as well as a result, of a *new line of questioning*, a philosophical contribution that issues in a new-found interiority.

Alternatively, spirituality, particularly as expressed in western tradition, is not just meditative exercises in search of the holy or an exploration of the mystery of *being*; it intends, also, to help an individual understand the temporality one lives with, as well as the need to resolve the burden of self-referential experiences. It does this through a series of spiritual exercises from meditation, to reflection, to self-understanding/mastery in order to experience self-forgetful *compassion* in our dealings with others and ourselves – dealings that are also marked by what we speak of as *justice*. It asks of those pursuing spiritual understanding that they encounter more directly, through a different history of questioning, the emptiness of the unlimited mist of possibilities that we have identified as the foundation for solitariness. A solitariness that we can depict as fully alive, a solitariness that grounds both psychoanalysis and spirituality, whose beingness can be grasped, paradoxically, only to the extent that we accept, as I have mentioned, its non-existence. I am not using these terms as some type of clever conundrum. Winnicott reminds us that, if we are dealing with the complexity of human beings, we have to accept paradox and not rush to resolve it or, one might add, to dismiss it out of intellectual frustration.

Perhaps the following image will help to clarify what I mean by a vital emptiness. Picture two large mirrors on opposing walls reflecting nothing but the space between them and consequently each other. We can, I believe, without too much violence to our topic, name one mirror psychoanalytic inquiry and the other mirror spiritual inquiry. And, for the sake of our analogy, we can name the empty space between them as the area of solitude, the ungraspable space of unlimited possibilities, out of which comes the quiet aloneness that makes both others and oneself real. Our analogy is somewhat weak, however, as psychoanalysis and spirituality are not existent realities in themselves;

they are a way of looking, a particular history of questioning, more like a certain angle at which we might place the mirrors to get a particular effect. And what they reflect is ultimately *nothing at all*. But, as mentioned, there is a profound paradox here because the nothing at all that we are speaking of is actually dense with possibilities made manifest in psychoanalysis through interpretations (meanings) and subsequent experiences and in spirituality through self-discipline and insight, as well as action.

To the extent that we appreciate the function of metaphors in organizing our conceptual world, we overcome the tendency to organize our experiences in terms of individuated, separate realities. Whitehead, as A. H. Johnson (1963) reminds us, calls such tendency in our thinking 'misplaced concreteness' (p. 150). Popularly speaking, we might say that human beings have an almost incurable attraction for missing the forest for the trees. Whitehead, however, thinks in terms of overriding operative principles that govern our experiences in the world. Such principles, somewhat akin to Plato's world of ideals, are more normative than the particular concrete objects that we encounter daily. To forget the interrelatedness of the world is to give individual objects a reality they cannot sustain; to appreciate the role of metaphor in our experience of knowledge is to perceive a wider and deeper world than specific concrete events. Winnicott's appreciation of metaphor and its role in life is reflected, as I mentioned above, in his understanding that an analysis can go on for years under the false assumption that the patient is alive – *alive* meaning, among other aspects, that a patient is able to play the play of metaphors. To be able to play with language is to understand metaphor rather than concreteness. It is from this viewpoint that I have spoken of psychoanalysis, as well as most spiritual traditions, each as a history of questioning, each with its own metaphors. Psychoanalysts speak of defenses, for example, whereas spiritual teachers speak of the discernment of spirits. Each particular history of questioning predetermines a particular response. Consequently psychoanalytic or spiritual truths can be only contextually validated, i.e., they are *made true* in context.[6] Each interpretation of symptoms, of actions, or of

---

6 Beller (1999) writing about the physicist Schrodinger notes 'the concept of reality' as such, 'as it objectively exists independent of all human observers, is indefensible, if not downright meaningless. Similarly, Schrodinger fully understood that the correspondence theory of truth can hardly be sustained. Still, the concept of reality, held Schrodinger, is as indispensable in science as it is in everyday life' (p. 282). I am in essential agreement with Schrodinger's thought.

unconscious factors is a unique creation that occurs between a particular analyst and a particular analysand; actually each interaction between analyst and analysand is a unique creation. Context, consequently, in its broadest meaning, helps us locate what is true for each individual. Therefore, 'understanding the metaphorical basis of knowledge frees us of the Herculean burden of finding the truth. We can, instead, settle for a truth, or should I say several truths' (Gargiulo, 1998a, p. 419). Truth, even contextual truth, deserves reverence, and an appreciation of metaphor serves that reverence. Dogma, psychoanalytic or spiritual, does not serve it well, because it attempts, in its misplaced concreteness, to quell anxiety by promoting a misguided narcissistic need to be the knowing other.

Several truths is another way of speaking, I would say, about a mist of unlimited possibilities, but unlimited possibilities in a different context, i.e., not in the nothingness of our inner being but in the functional actuality of our lives. Each patient ultimately has to find not only his or her way to aloneness, to solitude, but also his or her own way in the world. Winnicott's understanding that one essential facet of being alive is each person's need to create the found world is another way of saying this. This engagement is as equally true of the discipline of spiritual awareness as it is of psychoanalysis. Spiritual masters or teachers have the task of discerning the way; a psychoanalyst's task is not so different. The 'naming dialogue' of psychoanalysis is a struggle to *re-create* the world in the face of what we can call the *de-creation* of neurotic transference, in the face of the de-creation of what we identify as symptoms. Re-creation involves not just working through, with all that entails, but contacting the internal solitary ground from which our deepest sense of aliveness springs. An analyst's, as well as a spiritual master's, appreciation that there is no one correct path but rather only a mist of possibilities that *questioning* will either activate or not is the best guarantor of living with several truths. The psychoanalytic dialogue, consequently, echoes off the walls, so to speak, of both analyst and analysand, echoes off the non-existent seedbed of unlimited possibilities, and is heard in the solitary chambers of both. Within this context Winnicott's prayer, 'oh God, when I die, may I be alive' (Winnicott et al., 1989, p. 4), is not only strikingly psychoanalytic but profoundly spiritual as well.[7]

---

7 Anyone familiar with Zen thought or Vedantic Hinduism will hear echoes while reading Winnicott particularly, for example, in his understanding of the role of breathing in establishing a personal soma' (Gargiulo, 1998b, p. 154).

As we create our found world, we transform possibility into actual experience; we are then going from the everyday or natural transcendent to the historical immanent. Immanence in this context is the concretizing of particular possibilities, each interaction within the self and between the self and the other is a unique actualization, e.g., no two analyses can, or should be, the same. A patient with a different analyst has a different analysis. The same is true of spiritual discipleship. An everyday or natural transcendence, as I am using the term, reflects the awareness that possibilities, as such, are unlimited.[8] Such a definition allows us to de-sacralize the term transcendence without compromising its complexity.

So far I have followed the lead of Meister Eckhart, as well as the language of quantum mechanics, by blending what I have characterized as the emptiness of unlimited possibilities and relating it as foundational to the alone space of the individual, a solitariness that each individual negotiates throughout his or her life. When Eckhart prays, for example, 'to God that we may be free of God' (Colledge and McGinn, 1981, p. 200), he is attempting, I believe, to cross the perimeter into solitariness – past the language of sign signification (Colledge and McGinn, 1981). Eckhart's *God* is so radically different from traditional western usage that it is unfortunate he could not find another designation; given his time and place he had no choice.[9] When he implies, as I understand him, that to know oneself is to know the world, he is attempting to understand transcendence shorn of the concrete bifurcation that all too easily turns human beings and the world into an arena of objects to be managed.[10] What is ineffable in Eckhart's thought is what I would characterize as the unlimited possibilities of the solitariness of the world, so to speak. When he writes that one cannot even begin to know God unless one knows oneself, because to

---

8   Grotstein (2000) in *Who Is the Dreamer Who Dreams the Dream?* writes of the ineffable subject of the unconscious. When I speak of unlimited possibility that grounds existence, I am attempting to indicate a pre-subject mode out of which the *ineffable subject of the unconscious* can be spoken about. The ineffable subject is an actualization of transcendence giving birth to what psychoanalysts understand as the unconscious – an unconscious that, thanks to Grotstein's reading, is alive with meaning, with psychic presences. In terms of psychoanalytic understanding, Grotstein's notion of the ineffable subject captures what we can put into words. Eckhart speaks of the absolutely hidden and unknowable Godhead – for which even the term 'emptiness' seems too positive. The unlimited mist of possibilities is an attempt, given our language, to encompass both of these possibilities.

9   Note Eckhart's conviction that 'the greatest honor the soul can pay to God [is] to leave God to himself and to be free of him' (in McGinn, 2001, p. 145).

10 See Campbell (1986) for a discussion of such themes, particularly pp. 27–51.

know God is in some profound way to be God also, he is speaking, I believe, not as a religious missionary with a set of accepted formulas but as an individual who has struggled to put the non-existent quiet alone space of unlimited possibility into words.[11]

I have offered a personal reading of a few of the thoughts of this great mystic – thoughts that, as I have said, have little to do with convincing a person to believe but more to do with sensitizing a person to mystery, and to a sense of reverence for what grounds our life. If we practice psychoanalysis with correct technique but without a sense of mystery and reverence for each individual's solitary aloneness, we are wandering in a dark forest with no way out. 'We are poor indeed if we are only sane' (p. 150) was Winnicott's (1958) way of saying the same thing.[12]

Although spirituality is sometimes portrayed, by psychoanalysts, as the polar opposite of scientific, empirical thinking, its subject matter is, I have tried to show, not different from that of psychoanalysis. Spiritual traditions are of a different order, a different history of questioning than psychoanalysis, which fact, in itself, should not disqualify it as meriting thoughtful introspection. Spirituality, as it has developed in western societies, addresses the great silence within us. Spirituality has nothing to do with capturing that which cannot be captured; it is, I believe, a quiet response before the absolute silence of unlimited possibilities. Spiritual questioning, like psychoanalytic questioning, is made concrete, is made existent by actions. Overcoming the false import of the self, the narcissistic illusions of the 'I', is the foundation for sustainable self-awareness, for compassion, civility, and justice in our actions.

Such goals are actually common to both the psychoanalytic and the western spiritual traditions. The honesty Freud offers, when he proposed that we are not masters of our own house, has less to do with a deterministic philosophy than with promoting a muted sense of our own importance. The great aloneness that we all live with should engender a reverence for life. Reverence for life is an equal goal of psychoanalysis and of spirituality, a spirituality or psychoanalysis that

---

11 Note the following thought of Eckhart: 'The eye with which I see God is the same eye with which God sees me. My eye and God's eye is one eye and one seeing, one knowing, and one loving' (in McGinn, 2001, p. 149).

12 Note also Winnicott's (1988) statement 'I am doing nothing worse than I would do in saying of myself that I was sane and that through analysis and self-analysis I achieved some measure of insanity. Freud's flight to sanity could be something we psychoanalysts are trying to recover from' (p. 483).

has overcome self-aggrandizement. Only when we are alive, in Winnicott's meaning, can we experience compassion; only when we are alive are we comfortable with unknowingness; only when we are alive can we achieve a reverence for truth.[13] Such thoughts are not just the domain of spiritual writers; Francois Roustang, among other psychoanalysts, writes of similar concerns.[14]

In terms of each individual's 'historical actuality', in Erik Erikson's (1964, p. 206) sense, we have spoken of truth as contextual; in terms of our understanding of the profound emptiness that grounds human existence, we can speak of a non-contextual truth, if I can phrase it in such a manner – a truth that confirms that each human being is a momentary coming into being: each individual is an actualization of the natural transcendence of unlimited possibilities. We can think of that unlimitedness as the unconscious, the house of being, or the unspeakable, unknowable nothingness that grounds our lives.

Just as the psychological mechanisms of isolation, de-realization, or depersonalization have no place in a viable spirituality, so self-satisfaction, unreflective empiricism, and a lack of a capacity for civility and compassion have no place in a viable psychoanalysis. If an individual leaves analysis, as I have indicated, bereft of a profound sense of mystery, he or she is probably still suffering. If one enters the spiritual search bereft of a sense of the dark forest of our human pathologies, one is in danger of finding that one is living in a house without windows.

Human dignity is based on more than our functionality or our potentiality for meaningful actions; our dignity is based, as I have indicated, on an intuition that we somehow embody what is transcendent to the immediacy of our historical actuality. The psychoanalytic experience, its particular history of questioning, addresses the unlimitedness that not only grounds our lives but the equal unlimitedness with which we live. Psychoanalytic questioning is at a different

---

13 In a previous publication I noted: 'Terminating therapy, an individual should be able to love the world and to experience personal competence, to value themselves and be committed to the surprise of finding out who they are with honesty and humor. This is what it means to be alive. This is what it means to find oneself . . . We know our aloneness, however, because we are with others. Paradoxically when we are not in relation with others, we are not alone – we are isolated' (Gargiulo, 1999, pp. 344–345).

14 See Roustang (1982, 1983); both texts are dense with insight. Note, in particular, 'We conclude from the preceding argument that the cure is an act of inspired creation. The neurotic and even the psychotic are not suffering from too much imagination, but from too much reality. They are invaded by it because they dread it, and it freezes them in a repetitive process that prohibits the imagination from unfolding. Then come the permanent short circuits that doom the patient to sterility' (Roustang, 1983, p. 140).

angle, as we have depicted it, from spirituality, but it is clearly based on the same solitariness from which the histories of questions of spirituality arise. Psychoanalytic questions focus on transference, symptom resolution, and communication with our deepest creativity and spontaneity. Spiritual traditions speak of a discernment of spirits, a resolution of self-aggrandizing desire, and an invitation to touch the oneness of things – measured and reflected by one's mode of being in the world.[15] Psychoanalysis can lead to dead knowledge, most notably by a failure to foster the capacity to cross-identify. Spiritual exercises can fail to address narcissistic specialness, depersonalization, and/or schizoid isolation. Neither route, obviously, should be judged by its shortcomings or failures.

The awareness of the absolute aloneness of unlimited possibilities, which I have spoken of as a vital emptiness or nothingness, is the world – from a different view.

---

15 Discernment of spirits refers to a tradition wherein a person seeking spiritual counsel consults a recognized teacher who helps the student differentiate which practices and personal experiences can lead to spiritual enlightenment and which do not.

CHAPTER 3

Psychoanalysis, spirituality, and the possibility of meaning

Each experience in the world of events is what my identity constructs itself of . . .

William Kistler (1995, p. 74)

Since metaphors evoke a multitude of responses, it is rare, if even possible, for an author to know the full meaning of his or her work. This is certainly the case with Freud's creation of psychoanalysis: its richness is abundantly evident; his corpus is continually plumbed for insights. Whenever analysts or readers forget, however, that psychoanalysis is a creation and not a discovery and that metaphors are its scaffolding, its limitations also become evident. Freud believed, given his *conceptual* medicalization of psychoanalysis, that his new science discovered causes rather than uncovered possible/plausible reasons for psychological symptoms and/or experiences. In view of Wittgenstein's subsequent critique of psychoanalysis, however, we recognize that *causes* have to do with establishing empirical results; *reasons* are the psychological building blocks of self-awareness.[1] Meaning, as I use the term, is not primarily explanation; it has more to do with the exercise of self-awareness.

Freud, and his early followers, created an interpretative humanistic discipline, not an empirical science where possible causes are hypothesized and then tested. Psychoanalysis has not discovered any new ontological realities.[2] This is as true of Freud's initial topographical model as it is of his subsequent structural model: they are theoretical postulates. When an analyst suggests a cause for a particular action, symptom, or phantasy, he or she is proffering a reason, hopefully with as much circumstantial evidence as possible. Since a hundred different

---

1 For a comprehensive discussion of Wittgenstein's critique, see Bouveresse (1995, pp. 26–27).
2 Ontological, in this context, refers to realities that exist as individuated beings.

analysts, with a hundred different patients, offer different and, in many instances, effective interpretations of similar phenomena (they cannot be the same phenomena), it is clear that each analyst is offering a putative reason. When a patient is able to use such explanations, he or she will weave them into an overall tapestry of personal meaning and thereby gain further psychical integration, which is, ideally, the ability to resolve anxiety by experiencing more personal ownership of the events of one's life. Of course, all of the above is well known 100 years after psychoanalysis began to take shape.

The wide canvas of psychoanalysis not only encompasses an individual's psychological symptoms and offers a model for interpreting dreams but also attempts to analyze civilization itself, in its achievements, as well as its repressive aspects. Overall, it becomes evident that Freud, in fact, assumes a *Weltanschauung*, i.e., a system of belief that gives an interpretive framework for understanding the world. Given his nineteenth- century positivist education, Freud (1927) stands in the Apollonian tradition of reason and possibility of attaining truth. Note, for example, in *The Future of an Illusion*, when he writes that 'the voice of the intellect' (p. 53) will finally gain a hearing over illusion. Obviously, every system of thought reflects a particular *Weltanschauung*. The issue, consequently, is whether a particular world-view enables an individual to construct meaning within either an open or a closed system. Formulaic approaches are usually closed systems; they easily lend themselves to fundamentalist interpretations. It was against such closed systems of thought, exemplified for Freud by western religions, that he railed; he interpreted them as a flight from the demands of reality. But the line between a closed and an open system can be blurred, e.g., notwithstanding Freud's dismissal of religious beliefs, his insistence that the oedipal conflict is the universal causative complex for understanding psychoneurosis comes remarkably close to a closed system. That is what William James was alluding to when he characterized Freud as a man with *fixed ideas*.[3] We can, nevertheless, say that psychoanalysis is ultimately an open system, because it encourages alternative interpretations of life events, without punitive superego judgments. Such an approach fosters a personal individual experience of meaning rather than a collective experience. Whereas traditional western religious teachings, for example, focus on every individual's possession of free will and his or her consequent capacity to obey God-given dictates, Freud spoke of each

3 See John Kerr's (1994) *A Most Dangerous Method* (p. 245).

individual's graduated hard-won awareness and autonomy. The inherent tension between psychic determinism and autonomy was addressed by the English analyst Edward Glover (1963) when he spoke of the goal of therapy issuing in the capacity to experience *freed-will* (p. 193). Such a reading makes explicit the very rationale, or possibility, of psychotherapy, as well as a non-coercive experience of spirituality.

As psychoanalysis has matured it has deepened its understanding of the human situation, augmenting conflict resolution with the equally needed recognition for an individual to experience personal meaning. Meaning, in this context, does not entail imposing an overarching significance to one's life; it has more to do, I believe, with appreciating and personally integrating one's historical actuality. Meaning, in this context, is an active response to life's vicissitudes. Winnicott speaks of the child's need to create the found world, which, of course, is equally applicable to adults. *Creating the found world* is the capacity not only to *relate* to but also to *use* one's environment in a way that promotes personal growth. By personal growth I have in mind Winnicott's therapeutic and existential goal of being *alive*. Erik Erikson, for his part, speaks of the need to will the inevitable that has happened to one – another example, in his language, of integrating and using the world. Erikson's thought that one should be able to will the inevitable that has happened is an invitation to actively accept one's historical actuality and all the interdependence that such acceptance implies.

The construction of meaning entails a necessary dialogue with the unknown, i.e., a sensitivity to the depths of one's personal individuality, a depth that is, paradoxically, inextricably tied to the historical time in which one lives. This is the area of mystery in human experience. By the term 'mysterious' I mean an awareness of an ever-receding, yet simultaneously inviting, horizon to one's knowledge. Mystery does not entail a flight to a transcendent Other (God) who supplies truth and meaning to human existence. Whereas our social, cultural identity is of its very nature relational, and has its own dimension of mystery, an individual's experience of his or her essential solitariness, his or her essential aloneness, is the area that entails personal mystery. Winnicott, as we know, spoke of each individual's inviolable center of aloneness, a sacred area, which an analyst must never intrude upon. Religion, in Alfred North Whitehead's unique definition, 'is what one does with one's solitariness' (Whitehead, 1960, p. 16). Although not the commonly understood definition of religion, it is, nevertheless, a valid approach – an approach, I am aware, that has more to do with describing spirituality than religion. It is a definition that highlights the sacredness of the individual rather than the sacredness of the totally transcendent Other. Such a definition also avoids a closed system of thought; it allows for the possibility of what we can characterize as life-affirming spirituality in contradistinction to religious or dogmatic conformity. Spirituality, as I use the term, is one mode of addressing and experiencing one's individual solitariness, one's essential alone-ness. I say this because only by experiencing our essential aloneness, our solitariness, can we appreciate our deep connection with the world in which we live. It is only out of such an experience that we can learn to use the world, make it our own, and therefore experience meaning on an individual basis.

Most western spiritual traditions seek to promote the universal in the specific, i.e., enabling human beings to experience more of their profound interconnection with all life rather than focusing on the particularity of their own place and time. To contextualize this issue better, I would like to return to a concept I addressed in the previous chapter, namely what I have called the presence in human experience of an everyday transcendence.[4]

An everyday transcendence, as I have used the term, is an attempt to capture the awareness that we live in a world of infinite possibilities, from the micro to the macro level, a mist of infinite possibilities.[5] The awareness of a context of infinite possibilities makes any open system of thought possible. The human enterprise, as well as the world in which we live, is open-ended and constantly evolving. Paradoxically, and obviously, individuals are both limited and not limited by the con-creteness, i.e., the historical actuality, of their individual as well as collective histories. How one experiences one's personal subjectivity, one's essential aloneness, depends on the historical/cultural moment in which one lives, all of which affects the experience of meaning. Another way of saying this is to be aware that the language we speak

---

4 Anyone familiar with the works of James Grotstein will note, with my coining this term, my indebtedness.

5 Note Greene's (2000) definition of quantum determinism: 'Knowledge of the quantum state, however, determines only the *probability* [my italics] that one or another future will actually ensue' (p. 420). Insofar as the world of infinite possibilities is an ongoing creative concretiza-tion of probabilities, it exemplifies an aspect of what Whitehead (1957) postulates as God's consequent nature. Note Whitehead's thought: 'Neither God, nor the World, reaches static completion. Both are in the grip of the ultimate metaphysical ground, the creative advance into novelty' (p. 529). Whitehead, it is clear, does not subscribe to the metaphysical postulate of God's absolute otherness.

and hear informs the awareness we have about ourselves as well as of the world. The concept of an everyday transcendence is meant to suggest a pervasive ground to our daily experiences, out of which our creativity, our individuality as well as our culture grow.

Imagine, for a moment, each individual as an echo, so to speak, of a fuller voice. That fuller voice is an analogy for what we mean by an everyday transcendence, that area of the ever-inviting unknown, the area of mystery, which pervades life. One of the goals of therapy is to individualize, by giving personal adjectives, so to speak, to that fuller voice. Paradoxically, we can say that only out of an experience of encountering one's essential aloneness, the quiet mysterious depth of one's individual solitariness, can the experience of meaningful dialogue with the open-ended world begin.

Our psychoanalytic lens must, of necessity, get wider as we recognize that we live in a world of infinite possibilities, e.g., when analysts, artists, or poets interpret, they give form to the unformed mist of possibilities, they uncover a further horizon of mystery, and they create a new world in which to live. In psychoanalysis we create a new personal history, as Andre Green (1975) reminds us, a history not of illusion but of reconstructive interpretation. Paul Ricoeur (1970) was among the first philosophers of psychoanalysis to show that in analysis one has *a creative rendezvous* with one's personal history.[6]

Spirituality, as I use the term, is another way of approaching the human condition, another lens to interpret experience, to find the hidden in the present, a hidden that opens the present to a deeper appreciation of life. I do not believe it has to be inextricably tied to special states of consciousness or to any revelatory signs in the heavens above or the earth below. Like psychoanalysis, spirituality is an attempt to recognize and respond to the pervasive silence that surrounds and informs human life. Human beings are not deepened or expanded by the discovery of facts, be they the facts of one's history, one's defenses, and/or one's present life experiences. They are primarily motivated by a sense of and capacity to create meaning, which is a bridge to the personal and impersonal world in which we live. Such meaning makes both themselves and the world they live in inviting as well as mysterious. Ultimately, as we know, meaning must be personalized, it must have emotional as well as cognitive resonance for an individual, otherwise it is in danger of being experienced simply as a fact. Psychoanalysis, it bears repeating, is not an assimilation of psy-

---

6 See Ricoeur's *Freud and Philosophy* in Appendix A.

chological facts. *Where Id was, Ego will be,* of course, but as an essential consequence of that, we can add: to be humanly alive, to be real, means that we have a hand in creating the world we live in.

In trying to explain what I mean by creativity we might speak of each person as a *transparent mirror* (permit the contradiction for a moment). Such an image suggests that each person not only experiences the world as passing through and forming them, quite obviously, but also, and simultaneously, reflecting back and affecting, i.e., creating one's surroundings in response to what one is experiencing. When individuals look at a mirror, they see themselves as shaped by all that has happened to them. When the mirror is transparent, individuals are in contact with the world in which they live; they are a simultaneous response. Actually each human being is a point of reference, a temporary summation, for everything that has transpired in human history. We are not isolates unrelated to each other and/or to our world. We are not unconnected to each other; we, and the world we live in, are all made of the same *stuff.*[7]

Conceptualizing such a universal similarity is admittedly difficult. If we can picture, for a moment, human beings not simply as living on the Earth but being the Earth, in its consciousness – perhaps, being the cosmos itself, *in its awareness* – then my use of such categories as *mystery* or *spirituality* becomes, hopefully, more comprehensible. In using such an image as the *same stuff*, I am not suggesting a regression to an early oceanic merger with mother-world. The image of human consciousness as, perhaps, the Earth's awareness is a variant, I believe, of the Princeton physicist John Wheeler's strong anthropic principle.[8] Wheeler's thesis envisions the evolutionary emergence of humanity as central, i.e., causative, to the unfolding of the cosmos itself. If we can speak of the human psyche as somehow embodying or reflecting the Earth's consciousness, we also have another approach to understanding what we mean by the image of individuals as transparent mirrors. All of these considerations are in the service of gaining a fuller appreciation of our place in nature. The capacity to make sense of one's life, to bring a modicum of sense to what life itself is, depends on locating our experiences within as wide a context as possible. That

---

7 For a discussion of related themes see Corrington (1994, 1997). What I am attempting to address, with the image of the same stuff, is the inevitable narcissism that follows from conceptualizing human consciousness as simply and necessarily singular.

8 Compare Harrison (1981): 'The anthropic principle asserts that the universe is the way it is because we are here' (p. 287).

human consciousness itself comes out of the mist of infinite possibilities is the reason why we can speak of its openness to what I have called an everyday transcendence.

Only when we get past where we are can we know where we have been, which means, paradoxically, that in the moment we never know, definitively, where we are.[9] To be able to use the world, to create it by one's response to it, means to be able to tolerate a certain amount of not knowing where one is. What does such an open-ended approach imply for psychoanalytic practice or for spiritual understanding? Minimally it focuses on the element of surprise in one's experience with both oneself and the world. Personal meaning, as I have tried to delineate it, is an ever-renewing retrospective acceptance, as well as a creative use, of our experiences; consequently it allows for a not knowing in the present – for a non-dogmatic self-definition. Surprise is one of the rewards of creativity; what does not surprise us is ultimately boring. Surprise is one of the byproducts of metaphors, because metaphors mold significance out of the dull clay of facts that surround us.

Such an approach to the psychoanalytic dialogue is the ground space for clinical vitality. To be clinically vital is the opposite of compulsive ritualization of analytic technique. A lived appreciation of the metaphorical nature of knowledge helps avoid the pitfalls of such ritualization: a ritualization that all too frequently is characterized by a repetitive *figuring out* – a figuring out that seduces a practitioner into his or her head, instead of into his or her ears, which gives birth to psychological facts but is the opposite of the experience of meaning.[10] Creating the found world, creating personal meaning, it bears repeating, is not an exercise in figuring out life. Both patient and analyst look back to find and reconstruct their histories, although to reconstruct, I would suggest, has just as much to do with a person's history finding them.

Appreciating life on a deeper level than facts, appreciating existence itself and trying to grasp its import, has led many western thinkers to

---

9 Truth, as judgment, collapses awareness into time. In other words, if one could *be* in the moment simply with what *is*, we would experience truth without having to be aware of it, i.e., without having to make a judgment.

10 Obviously we can say that in order to understand we have to figure things out. More to the point, however, is the reality that in order to understand we have to get past figuring out. To learn anything we have to transcend it – we have to get beyond it, otherwise we cannot know it.

speak of a *ground*, an organizing framework by which to know the world. From the medieval Meister Eckhart, who spoke of the ground as the *absolute unnamable*, to the modern German philosopher Martin Heidegger (1966, 1977), who finds the ground in the *unconcealment of being*, as well as to Freud, who reads the *unconscious* as ground enough, we have reason to posit that there is more to our knowledge than we can grasp. Such is the area I have spoken of as *mystery*; such is, for example, what the term *unconscious* points to, which the phrase *everyday transcendence* attempts to capture – the echo that we personalize or, we could also say, is personalized through us. *Ground* obviously implies, as well as gives birth to, a multi-dimensionality of meanings.[11] What we have designated as a world of infinite possibilities, which is a metaphor for the world we experience as totally open-ended, addresses the same issue.

Psychoanalytic findings have made us aware that any belief has to be examined by experience, and experience has to be constantly questioned in order to know what it is. A capacity for mystery and awe, in the sense that I use these terms, is consequent upon an examination of experience; it is not a substitute for it. Freud overemphasized rational analysis and downplayed mystery. Winnicott (1958) addressed this shortcoming when he noted that 'we are poor indeed if we are merely sane' (p. 150) and indicated that psychoanalysis had to recover from Freud's flight to sanity (compare Winnicott et al., 1989, pp. 482–492). A capacity to experience mystery in our lives prepares us to hear more than what we can ever anticipate.

Not only has psychoanalysis freed us from moralistic superego constraints, it is a new moment, a new turn, in human awareness. In its ability to address the repetitive patterns of one's past and resolve pernicious narcissism, which ultimately isolates human beings, it can be characterized as fostering spiritual enlightenment. It can serve as a meeting place, so to speak, out of which we can give birth to our world, just as the world gives birth to us. This is so because psychoanalysis universalizes individual experiences as it individualizes universal experiences. Consequently we can say that each life is obviously one's own and not one's own – *not one's own* because each person is shaped by culture, molded by language, and formed by parents. Desire, that perennial demi-urge of the psyche, has many

---

11 For many people throughout the world, belief in a monotheistic God is their ground. Albert Einstein spoke of an experience of awe as his sensitivity to something beyond the human but not definable.

incarnations, only one of which, transference, has psychoanalysis explored with any focused intensity. But, if we are going to speak about the need to personally create the found world, we have to complement the potentially distorting aspects of transference desire with that which we can characterize as relational desire.[12] By this I mean that arena of human desire that attempts to capture our yearning, as well as our need, for each other in ways other than the unrecognized or repressed demands of body and/or personal history. Relational desire ties our internal world to the external world.

Creating meaning from the tumble of facts that make up our lives brings us to a more basic and paradoxical position, however, i.e., no discussion of personal meaning is possible, I believe, without addressing, even in a most cursory manner, what the individual 'I' means – the 'I' with which we are singularly comfortable, as well as the 'I' that is simultaneously elusive and mysterious – the 'I' that is our own, the 'I' that is not our own. When our sights are on that 'I' with which we are comfortable, psychoanalytic insights have been particularly helpful; when our sights are on the 'I' that is elusive and mysterious, we cross over to the land that mystery, poetry, and spirituality explore.[13] I continue this discussion in Chapter 4.

To interpret unconscious content and/or processes is one example of *creating the found world* in which we live. If we borrow, again, some findings from quantum mechanics, we can say that observation determines results. Or we can likewise say that the questions we ask determine the answers we get. The unconscious, which is the psychoanalytic gateway to what grounds human experience, is a product of our observation, because what we give form to is ultimately a concretization out of the world of infinite possibilities in which we live. That there are many worlds that can be given form makes any commitment to one world less absolute, but also less relative.

That the psyche, in all its complexity, despite its dark manifestations, can be conceptualized as the Earth's self-awareness offers the possibility of freeing us from the narcissism of our own singularity, so to speak, a narcissism that both psychoanalysis and spiritual traditions have, on occasion, contributed to. Ideally, both spiritual paths and psychoanalytic experience should enable an individual not only to have a capacity for psychological insight but also to experience civility,

---

12 For a more detailed discussion of relational desire, see Chapter 6.
13 In this vein I am reminded of the poet Borges' (1999) lines when he writes, 'if, in fact, I am an I' (p. 93).

self-forgetfulness, vulnerability, and compassion. Each of the separate, yet related, routes of psychoanalysis and/or spirituality can prepare us for a more communal experience of life, an experience where the distinction between what is psychoanalytic and what is spiritual need not be asked.

Finally we can say that, if in order to know anything we have to get beyond it, to experience personal meaning we have to, paradoxically, transcend it. Erikson (1963, p. 268 et seq.) suggests as much when he speaks of ego integrity and wisdom and our need to pass our insights onto the next generation, quietly yet acutely aware of the relativity of those insights. Human subjectivity needs to be appreciated as both singular and collective, internal and simultaneously external; each individual (and culture) is a momentary concretization within the generic background of a mist of infinite possibilities. As we create the world we live in, new worlds open to us.

In Chapter 4, I revisit our understanding of the unconscious, as well as our notion of an 'I', to see if we can free these concepts from the non-metaphorical worlds in which they have sometimes functioned.

Mind, metaphor, and the 'I' in psychoanalysis and spirituality

Natural science . . . describes nature as exposed to our method of questioning . . . it makes the sharp separation between the world and the I impossible.

Werner Heisenberg (1999, p. 81)

. . . the multiplicity and differences that distinguish individuals are likewise but appearances.

Goethe (in Campbell, 1986, p. 113)

In this chapter I would like to address further the concepts of *mind* and *the autonomous 'I'* within both the psychoanalytic and western spirituality traditions.

Psychoanalysis, I have argued, mirrors, in its inquiry into personal meaning and in its efforts to achieve integration and reconciliation, similar issues to those addressed within spirituality traditions, with the exception, of course, of belief in a transcendental theistic reality.[1] Although psychoanalysis does not address such a reality, it does concern itself with an individual's experience of being alive, of living creatively in the world with others, and of finding some modicum of personal meaning beyond the mere facts of one's life. Many spirituality traditions do likewise. To better ground psychoanalytic and spirituality similarities, I focus primarily on two concepts that form the bedrock of psychoanalytic reflections, i.e., the idea of the autonomous 'I', and the concept of mind. These are, quite obviously, complex topics. My intention is simply to open up a line of inquiry in order to situate the discussion.

---

1 To understand the past (an essential task of psychoanalysis) is ultimately to forgive the past; more specifically, in Erik Erikson's thoughts, maturation is evidenced by a capacity to will the inevitable that has happened to us.

Before psychoanalysis spoke of the need for object constancy in its understanding of how we function as integrated persons, Meister Eckhart addressed the experience of personal individual internality and communal externality. He taught, following in a philosophical tradition that had its roots in ancient Greece, that each person is not an isolate but interconnected to all that is.[2] He understood that to know oneself is to know the world and to know the world is to know oneself. Eckhart employed a theological language that is known as *the negative way*, i.e., a theology that recognizes the anthropocentric quality of any God talk and, consequently, the need to speak less about any theistic reality and to experience more of what gives life meaning, in the here and now. Although a medieval Christian theologian, he was able to reflect that it would be more religious to imitate Jesus than to worship him.[3] A grounded mystic, Eckhart spoke of living a life of compassion and consideration for others, of listening to the deep silence that is within us in order to hear the silence of the other and of the world. Most contemporary democratic societies, although using different language, echo such sentiments; they recognize, at least in theory if not always in practice, that all life is to be valued, and that each person is to be respected and promoted in his or her life goals. Within the psychoanalytic tradition Winnicott, in particular, has focused on the therapeutic, as well as life-goal, for an individual to feel alive, to experience life as a self-fulfilling creative arena rather than a journey leading nowhere.

Psychoanalysis, in its commitment to addressing defenses, in its desire to help people live in the present, free of the troubling past and the elusive future, would have little difficulty in embracing many of Eckhart's thoughts. One need not accept the range of Eckhart's Christian beliefs in order to recognize that he found and explored a profound depth of human experience – not unlike psychoanalysts, who are midwives of meaning, explorers, with their patients, in their search for personal depth. It is in this sense that we can speak of psychoanalysts as true heirs to western spiritual traditions. They are guides helping their patients discern what is true from what is no longer true, real from all that is not real, what is the now from all that has passed away. They are healers who are both scientific and spiritual in their goals: scientific, in limiting the range of inquiry with an openness to alternate viewpoints and formulations, and spiritual, in the desire to

---

2 Such teaching reflects early Stoic beliefs.
3 That there is a bridge between Eckhart's thought and Buddhism is clear; see, for example, Merton (1968) and Fromm et al. (1960).

find a truth for a given life beyond the recurrent distortions and defensive reactions that cloud such a possibility.

Now to examine some basic concepts about the mind, and the autonomous 'I'.

Winnicott's (1958) perceptive article 'Mind and its relation to the psyche- soma' suggests that mind, as a localizable thing, does not exist. Always interested in context, he speaks about 'mental activity as a special case of the functioning of the psyche/soma' (p. 254).[4] Winnicott complements these thoughts when he writes of the transitional space of childhood being the seedbed of culture. In writing of the child's developmental stages of me/not me experiences with the early mother/other/environment, he lays the foundation for our human capacity to play with the world and thus to create culture. Building on such reflections, one can speak of mind, I suggest, as best exemplified in humanity's cultural achievements, i.e., we come to know mind through all the languages of culture. It is, consequently, not reducible to a biological entity. Consciousness, which is uniquely dependent on neurological brain functioning, is a prerequisite for the experience of mind, but it is not co-equal. Consciousness, in human experience, makes the awareness of mind possible. But meaning, which is the calling card of mind, so to speak, is singularly a communal accomplishment – within such a framework we can say that to speak of culture is to speak of mind.[5] And, quite obviously, to speak of culture is to speak of a gestalt. Dr Lewis Thomas (1974), struggling with similar thoughts, uses the image of looking down on a giant anthill as an analog of human cultural activity. Concurrently, if we speak of mind as evidenced in the works of our cultural (communal) hands, so also, I believe, can we speak of our sense of self, i.e., our experience of our 'I', as arising within and reflecting a particular cultural setting. Just as Winnicott could write, now rather obviously, that there is no such thing as a baby (without a mothering environment) so can we say that the 'I' does not exist, singularly, in itself. By *singularly* I mean out of the context of understanding the 'I' as a cultural/imaginative construct, as a metaphor for the experience of the self as social. What I mean by that is best captured by the paradox of the self as social and relating to the culture in which it functions, as well as being formed by and therefore identifiable within that very culture. Of course by saying this I have not

---

4 For a contemporary approach to this issue, see *Looking for Spinoza*, by Antonia Damasio (2003).

5 For an extensive and insightful discussion of this topic, see Cavell (1988).

said anything new. Individuals are the crossroads of biology and culture.[6] The 'I' that faces the world and that experiences its own inner world knows itself through the culture into which it is born.[7]

Western European culture has emphasized the autonomous self, the individual as a self-contained 'I' – not without some justification, I am aware. Such an approach needs to be counterbalanced, however, by appreciating the 'I' as a product of a particular culture – understanding that the commonality of our human experience means that each 'I' is a moment of, and therefore a product of, cultural evolution. The obvious paradox here needs to be sustained if we wish to appreciate the respective contributions of psychoanalytic thought and/or spiritual/ philosophical insights.[8]

If the goal of psychoanalysis can still be thought of as one's ability to love and to work, we are immediately in the arena of the other – the other who creates desire, the other, of culture, who molds identity. This does not obliterate what we refer to as the 'I' – it simply locates its metaphorical base. The 'I' is like a mirror reflecting both inner and outer worlds. The emphasis on intrapsychic structures, as if there is a separate entity, an ontological 'I', has been misleading and dangerous in its consequences; it has promoted an exaggerated notion of personal autonomy. Autonomy is the experience of competence within a particular culture, a culture that gives individuals a language by which to name both themselves and the world they inhabit.

Psychoanalysts name and give voice to the varied aspects of personal identity, their own and their patients'; in doing so, they situate an individual within a particular cultural framework. From this perspective the analytic process mirrors the family, just as the family mirrors society, in its defining functions for the individual. Twentieth-century philosophy has helped us appreciate that language forms consciousness, just as consciousness forms language, i.e., we are formed by the language that is spoken to us, a language not only of words but also

---

6 I am aware that I am using the terms 'self' and 'I' interchangeably. Self has a wider meaning, encompassing the subjective mapping of bodily functions whereas the 'I', as I am using the term, refers to a particular content of consciousness – consequently my thought that it is an imaginative/cultural construct.

7 Speaking to this issue, the philosopher Francis Jacques (1991) writes: 'Both empirical subjectivity and the status of person are derived from subjectivity sometimes as an effect, sometimes as an illusion, but never as a basic principle.' (I think the concept of illusion is misleading; it suggests a phantasy in contradistinction to an imaginative construct, which, as I have tried to show, implies engagement with the culture one inhabits.)

8 That the emphasis in western cultures, in particular, on autonomous individuality is consonant with a capitalistic economy should not be lost sight of.

of meanings, a language that helps individuals know and map their internality. We have to be repeatedly called by a name, repeatedly told we are an autonomous 'I', for us to be able to organize our experience in such a category. How we are called by and within our culture commits us to what we hear about ourselves and about our world. Nor do we have a choice; such a process is the way we pass on cultural patterning.

Psychoanalysis looks for the hidden in the obvious, for an alternative meaning behind the manifest meaning. From such a perspective, one would have expected psychoanalysis to be a radical critique, following Fenichel and some of the early analysts, of society's identifying processes. Why this did not occur has been discussed by Russell Jacoby (1983) and cannot detain us here, but the question as to whether psychoanalysis should address the cultural product of the 'I' should concern us, even in a preliminary, cursory way.

One of the difficulties in the task of correcting the distortions of the overemphasis on *the autonomous 'I'* is, I believe, related to Freud's theoretical conceptualizations of the early vicissitudes of narcissism. As a point of reference and reflection, Freud speaks of the infant as possessing both primary and secondary narcissism. Primary narcissism, as a postulate for the life force holding together and fostering growth, is an understandable postulate. Secondary narcissism, as the capacity of a young infant to withdraw libido from the other, from the outside world and invest it in the self, is more than misleading. It is misleading because there is no *self* except in the context of another. Freud assumes what he is trying to prove, namely that the self is *self-contained*, as if there is a separate operational 'I' directing the flow of libidinal investments. But libidinal investments are always a context experience (i.e., child/mothering/environment). A child, or an adult, can imagine that he or she has withdrawn interest from the world, but this results in what Winnicott refers to as split-off intellect, i.e., *mind*, thought of as located in a thing we call the brain. Unfortunately, without an adequate parental environment supporting a young infant, he or she can easily start on the road of such splitting from that environment, with the concurrent illusion that he or she is a separate entity – an 'I' unto him- or herself.

The mothering person is defined by his or her caring for the child's developing physical needs and concurrent language/social/emotional needs. If that individual mix-up of mutual needs and services goes well enough, both the caretaker and cared for have an experience of being alive in their bodies without experiencing themselves as locked in their heads. Given a positive early environment, the cultural transmission of oneself, as an 'I', can be experienced as primarily relational and interdependent, and not simply as separate and autonomous. One of the indications that a relational and interdependent self is present is an individual's capacity to experience cross-identification, the ability to put oneself in another's shoes, so to speak. Is such a capacity what Winnicott intends when he says that were we able to raise children with good enough environmental provision there would be no need to teach them morality, they would have a natural ethics? We are, to repeat, an 'I' in context; this in no way, however, obviates our biological substratum. What it does indicate is that language, as I have mentioned, uses us and defines us as much as we use it. Further, without a cultural context, our drives cease to be human drives and become merely physical sensations. To love and to work, as Freud knew, means infinitely more than negotiating physical sensations. Within this context we can note that instincts do not have vicissitudes, people do.

Another difficulty in the path for analysts to fully appreciate the import of an interdependent and relational 'I' has been the traditional psychoanalytic understanding of the unconscious. With Freud's introduction of the structural model, the unconscious went, so to speak, from being a noun to being an adjective; it persisted, nevertheless, in being thought of as somehow *located* in a person, individually, i.e., as if it had individual ontological status. Obviously, there is a great deal that human beings do not know about themselves, and still more that they do not want or wish to know about themselves. Such is the human condition, and psychoanalysis, in particular, has brought such awareness to the forefront and speaks of it as repression. Freud's move, however, from the topographical to the structural model was not simply a recognition of the ego's role in defenses but was also a move away, I believe, from concretizing the unconscious.

Explicit in Freud's thinking was the conviction that we can recognize what we have turned our psychological eyes away from through dialogue, either personal or interpersonal. Language pre-eminently gives form to, and in that sense creates, awareness. Freud's topographical model of the unconscious can still be useful, nevertheless, but it would then refer to what I have characterized as the solitary depth of the individual, the alive emptiness that I spoke of in Chapter 2 – a vital emptiness that is both personal and transcendent. Such emptiness, which I have spoken of as a world of infinite possibilities, is constantly coming into being, is constantly created and given form by our experience of it, by our naming it. We can analogously compare what I mean by *creating* the unconscious *by interpretation* to what quantum mechanics speaks of when it notes that a particular experiment confirms a particular premise, e.g., do we want to observe light as a wave or a particle? Each hypothesis can be demonstrated by how the experiment is structured. The works of our individual and cultural hands are always creating, and are always, consequently, giving form to the unconscious.[9] (For the present discussion I leave aside the question of unconscious thinking, defenses, or motivation.)

As mind can be approached as manifesting itself in the experience of culture, as communal, its reality cannot be split off from that communality. Meaning, as I have indicated, is as culture bound as is the autonomous 'I'. Both can be approached as imaginative cultural constructs. By imaginative constructs I intend to point to the personal elaborations, the personal schemas we bring in response to cultural constructs, to formative cultural influences. The reading of any text, and here I include both dreams and symptoms, is dependent on the cultural framework of the reader. An analyst's interpretative reading of an unconscious component is primarily one of many possible interpretations. Consequently, we can say that analyst, patient, and culture join together to create the mind out of which come particular interpretations. Speaking to this issue, the philosopher Jacques (1991, p. 297) notes:

> Let us therefore remember the dialogical principle: an utterance is produced in a community of meaning, in some way bilaterally, between utterers who interact, bivocally, through dual listening and meaning.

Without interpretation we do not know what we experience. Human thoughts and actions are complex because they are open to alternative readings, i.e., we are capable of generating and understanding metaphor. That we can think metaphorically means that interpretations are potentially endless.

Psychoanalysis has come to appreciate that there is more to life than the resolution of neurotic conflict; it is, in fact, the capacity to find life interesting and worthwhile by experiencing ourselves as connected with the world, not isolated in our own thinking, creative in our interactions,

---

9 I am *not* speaking, in this context, of Jung's universal archetypes.

and not simply reactive to our environment. Cultural experiences and individual experiences are inextricably related, so much so that mind does not exist as a *localized thing*, primarily because it is a process that occurs between people, between self and other, *as other and as cultural world*. Such an approach does no violence, I repeat, to our personal psyche/soma experiences of memory, thought, and imagination. If mind does not exist as a localizable thing, to follow Winnicott's lead, it nevertheless resides in all the cultural bridges we have built: language, art, philosophy, religion, and psychoanalysis, to name just a few. To all appearances the Earth is stable, just as to all appearances we are autonomous I's and our minds are talked about as if they are individual personal possessions. Such perceptions are correct as well as misleading. The Earth is stable, but not static, it is moving all the time. Likewise we can certainly say that we have a personal 'I', seemingly autonomous; on closer examination, however, this perception does not tell the whole story. Likewise we can say that the psyche is personal, but mind is communal and belongs to culture. We walk on bridges; our very coming to be is a bridge experience. When Winnicott says, for example, that the first thing a patient should be able to do is play, he is talking about getting someone off an illusory island and onto a bridge; getting someone out of the house of mirrors of the anxious ego (mind and 'I' as pathological isolates) and into the marketplace of life.

Herbert Fingarette (1963), in his *The Self in Transformation*, made analysts aware that their primary goal was the resolution of the anxious ego, which then makes possible a sensible living in the now of time and the here of space. To experience our interdependence, familial and cultural, is not only realistic; it resolves the illusion that one has an 'I' that is definable in itself. Within such a framework, psychoanalysis mirrors spiritual traditions which have as their operational goals an individual's capacity for communal civility (i.e., cross-identification) rather than schizoid isolation, unencumbered personal presence rather than neurotic repetition, love that sees the other as such, not as a mirror, or a mother, and, finally, work that is done competently but not necessarily self-consciously. Cross-identification does not entail obliterating the differences of the here and now of one's existence. Rather, it develops as one is able to recognize the relativity and therefore the commonality of the 'I'. Such recognition fosters a willingness to entertain differences in time, place, and cultural identity. To recognize our commonality with others, via resolution of the narcissism of the anxious ego, is, as we have mentioned, a hoped-for outcome of the analytic process. Desire, which is integral to an understanding of the 'I', can be understood, as I have noted elsewhere, as transference desire (repetitive self-preoccupation) or relationship desire (see Gargiulo, 1989). I discuss relationship desire in Chapter 5; for now, however, we can note that in naming desires, both manifest and latent, psychoanalysis provides for their partial integration. Partial because desire, similar to the 'I', is not a solitary experience; it is not rooted only in our biological substratum but is also created and augmented by the other, and by the culture, family, and society in which one lives.

T.S. Eliot (1943, p. 36), in *Little Gidding*, speaks to such issues:

This is the use of memory:
For liberation – not less of love but expanding
Of love beyond desire, and so liberation
From the future as well as the past.

Psychoanalysis, freed from the bifurcation of subject and object, offers the possibility for understanding a spirituality that is humanly possible rather than religiously necessary – a liberation, which Eliot alludes to, that is, in fact, more of an ongoing task than an actual accomplishment, a liberation that, in experiencing the interconnection of self and other, of past, of present, and, of necessity then, future, provides, paradoxically, for the possibility of living more deeply in the ever-elusive now.

Augustine, long before Freud, advocated that we should 'love, and do what you will' (in Przywara, 1958, p. 341), meaning, I believe, that a person only finds, and in that sense creates him- or herself, with and through others. That psychoanalysis reminds human beings of the normative and formative role of love is particularly well stated in Jonathan Lear's (1990) *Love and Its Place in Nature*. As we are listened to, we know that we have a voice; as we are cared for, we know that we can love the world. As we construct meaning and culture, mind and the 'I', as we appreciate self and other, we are, in fact, loving the world. From such a perspective, is there much difference in the goals of psychoanalysis or of a viable spirituality?

CHAPTER 5

Authority, the self, and psychoanalytic experience[1]

Desire itself is movement
Not in itself desirable;
Love is itself unmoving
Only the cause and end of movement,
Timeless and undesiring.

T.S. Eliot (Four Quartets, 1943, p. 8)

In this chapter I would like to discuss some of the issues implicit in the traditional philosophical categories of subject and object, and the psychoanalytic parallel: the self and the other. I discuss the *self* and the experience of autonomy, and the *other* and the experience of authority. These are discussed in terms of two unifying references, namely transference desire and relationship desire. I would like to suggest a broadening of psychoanalytic discourse to enable a better appreciation of the subject–object distinction. To do this we first have to raise a core question: Is there a hermeneutics to human desire? Such a question entails more than is encompassed by the traditional Freudian postulate that there is teleology to human instinctuality.

Paul Ricoeur (1981), in *Hermeneutics and the Human Sciences*, states: 'Hermeneutics is the theory of the operations of understanding in their relation to the interpretation of texts' (p. 43). Therefore, to speak of a hermeneutics of human desire is to employ an analog, i.e., human desire is approached as if it were a (complicated) literary text, perhaps best exemplified in the form of poetry. Rather than speak of truth or error, in an unreflected way, we can address the area of discourse that an author employs and the specific issues addressed within that area. To accomplish this we should know the models a particular

---

1 This chapter is a slightly revised version, under the same title, of an article that appeared in The Psychoanalytic Review (1989).

writer employs as well as the operative metaphors in which those models are used.[2] It is important not only to know the questions being raised but also to appreciate that commensurate with given questions there is an inherent limitation on any possible answers. Heisenberg (1999, p. 58) addresses this point when he notes:

> . . . we have to remember that what we observe is not nature itself, but nature exposed to our method of questioning. Our scientific work in physics consists in asking questions about nature in the language that we possess and trying to get an answer from experiment by the means that are at our disposal.

Contrast, for example, Freud's intrapsychic structural model (id, ego, superego) with Winnicott's maturational object relations model (i.e., the human self as developmentally relational – finding and creating the found world). Such diverse models enable us to experience (and therefore to interpret) the reality under observation differently. Freud (1905) stated that in studying instinct he was primarily tracing the vicissitudes of the psychical instinctual representative, whereas Winnicott (1965) makes it clear that he intends to study, in his approach to man, the space, both actual and potential, between the *me* and the *not me*.

Ricoeur (1970), re-formulating the concept of a dynamic psychic tension, which Freud's structural model addressed, speaks about desire having a rendezvous with authority. I use the term 'desire' to indicate that area of human experience, somewhere between developmental maturational needs, that cannot be negotiated without serious consequences for personal development, and infantile (hallucinatory) wishes that will not be negotiated, i.e., childhood demandingness. For example, the experience of self-respect is a crucial developmental need, whereas excessive narcissistic self-reference is an all-too-human (infantile) wish. Desire connotes wish, although it should not be unreflectedly equated with instinctuality. In childhood, personal instinctual wishing is tied to the gratifying and/or depriving available parental object, who is, in fact, developmentally necessary for growth. The parenting figure's appropriate response to the child's needs is the seedbed for a person's experience of self-respect. Relationship desire is therefore grounded developmentally in a different experience from

---

2 I use the term 'operative metaphors' to point to those personal and cultural presuppositions and modes of thought that organize reality and our experience of it.

instinctual transference desire. Transference desire arises all too frequently when parents have not resolved their own narcissistic self-referential proclivities and thus aggravate the child's dependency on them by stimulating his or her own anxious self-reference. Thus, they augment an emotional misperception of the role of the other (and the self) in satisfying basic human needs. Returning to Ricoeur's phrase 'desire has a rendezvous with authority', we can note that authority means the other, the powerful other. That this authority is, in actuality, both transferentially and relationally experienced (given the present state of parenting) is one of the more serious complications in human growth. This is so because authority mediates and focuses the experience of personal desire. When this desire is a product of an (anxious) ego, under the spell of self-reference, it represents transference wish, i.e., it distorts the experience of the other, as traditional analytic clinical experience has abundantly shown.

To understand relational desire, we need simply reflect on the fact that a person is made structurally interdependent with his or her caretakers not only by early developmental experiences, but also by the very processes that make human self-consciousness possible, or, in a word, language. Human beings are bound in cross-identificatory processes of desire; cross-identification means that one sees oneself in the face of the other.[3] Human beings yearn for recognition. We want (desire) the other and we desire the other's desire of us. The other binds desire, i.e., the other makes the experiencing subject aware of desire:

> We can then understand one of Lacan's celebrated formulations: the unconscious is the discourse of the Other. By his speech, which evokes, desires, or prohibits, the Other stamps memories with the seal of pleasure and stamps events forced out of memory with the seal of shame or suffering.
>
> Vergote (1983)[4]

Thus, both object (the other) and subject (the self) are integral to desire. One cannot speak, consequently, of instincts solipsistically, as if they were comprehensible in themselves, as if source and/or aim was the only essential consideration, or as if transference desire encompassed the totality of human desire.[5] In fact Winnicott speaks

---

3 This is a modification of Freud's notion of the ego as the precipitate of past cathexis.
4 Note also Lacan's (1977) observation: 'man's desire is the desire of the Other' (p. 312).
5 This obviously has implications for psychoanalytic technique. Note Musud Khan's (1975, pp. xi–xlviii) observation that many of the classic technical interventions cause the very resistances that the technique is designed to overcome.

of instincts being psychologically meaningful only within the context of the experience of personhood. As a child negotiates such developmental needs as the experience of self-respect and personal recognition, cross-identification becomes a cornerstone for relational desire which bridges the distance between the self and the other.

When the analyst asks for the patient's associations, he or she is trying to grasp the context in which and by which to understand the patient's communication. To look at a society's associations, so to speak, we must study the operative myth models so as to understand the individual within that society as well as the society at large. Particular myth formulations/structures are the context out of which particular personal/cultural and intellectual metaphors take their meaning. As desire, both individually and collectively, takes place within the context of a particular myth model, we have to appreciate this fact in any hermeneutic study of desire, i.e., self-experience and perception of the world are both organized by the operative scientific and cultural myth models that mediate desires and, in fact, make desires known to the self.[6] Consequently perception may be thought of as a function of personal desire (both transference and relational) as mediated through a particular historical/cultural tradition. We see what we *desire* to see, and we see what our *culture enables* us to see.[7]

This is elucidated in Winnicott's (1958, pp. 229–242) transitional object model, i.e., we do not simply find the objective world we live in; we create it by giving it meaning. Or, more specifically, note Winnicott's (1971) approach to play – not the play of games but of two people entering that in-between place of the me/not me, creating a shared world of imagination and/or discourse. For his part, Freud created psychoanalysis through the questions he asked, and he asked these questions based on the metaphors available to him. Dreams, for example, became psychoanalytically meaningful as a result of his topographical model. What we know of the world is largely what we allow ourselves to know. (Similarly, what an analyst knows of a patient is, in good part, what he or she allows him- or herself to know.) Italo Calvino (1974) informs us that 'It is not the voice that commands the

---

6 Good mothering, for example, as Erikson (1963) has made clear, is highly contextualized by the cultural metaphors available to the mother. This refers not only to the content of mothering but also to the very desire for mothering.
7 For an interesting discussion of such a perspective, see Gerhardi (1981).

story: it is the ear' (p. 106).[8] Yet the voice attracts the ear to listen, just as a mother's response evokes desire in the child. Winnicott accepts this paradox when he observes that the objective mother is waiting to be created by the child. The mother, as the foundation for the subsequent use of transitional objects, serves as a necessary bridge to/for the child finding and creating the object, objectively perceived, which is the other.

Following Winnicott, we may note that creativity takes place in the transitional space between the subjectively real and the object objectively perceived. This object objectively perceived is, as we have noted, subject to the models we employ to experience both personal (subjective) desires and the world (the objective other) desires. Another example of operative myth models and human experience may be seen in the works of Whitehead. Whitehead (1960) posits normative principles, e.g., creativity, as necessary postulates for knowing reality.[9] Consequently, in the area of epistemology, he concludes that most knowledge exemplifies what he terms 'misplaced concreteness'. By misplaced concreteness, Whitehead means that we take for an object of scientific observation what appears to our senses as an object in itself separable from the whole context of its occurrence. Whitehead considers all western philosophy to be a footnote to Plato and, although he does not postulate an ideal world, he argues persuasively that humans have a consistent habit of missing the forest for the trees. In psychoanalytic discourse we would speak about limiting perception to manifest content (misplaced concreteness) while ignoring latent meaning.

By way of interim conclusion we can note the following: without an appreciation of the reality of and distinction between transference desire and relational desire, and the search for the powerful other, without the awareness that humans create the world in order to perceive it (myth model), and without a critical appreciation of the ever-present possibility of misplaced concreteness, psychoanalysis would, in effect, be a nineteenth-century Newtonian psychology or, in other words, a given world that has fixed points of reference, in

8 A literary description of the elusiveness of any objective reality vis-à-vis our desires is beautifully summarized by Calvino: 'At this point Kublai Khan expects Marco to speak of Irene as it is seen from within. But Marco cannot do this: he has not succeeded in discovering which is the city that those of the plateau call Irene. For that matter, it is of slight importance: if you saw it, standing in its midst, it would be a different city; Irene is a name for a city in the distance, and if you approach, it changes' (Calvino, 1974, p. 99).

9 For a perceptive exposition of Whitehead's thought, see Johnson (1963).

contradistinction to the *relative* (point of reference) world that both Einsteinian and quantum mechanics have made available to us.[10]

In the Freudian tradition, the self and the other are experienced through the model of transference (desire). In this paradigm, transference reflects our constant proclivity to relive the past in the present, and entails, within the psychoanalytic setting, the interplay of reciprocal fantasies and desires. 'Desire is interplay; transference is interplay' (Roustang, 1982, p. 56).[11] Thus, the classic presumption: desire is transference. This is so, I would add, when desire is not related to developmental needs but arises from the narcissistic (anxious) ego. From the Freudian perspective, limiting desire to transference desire creates the ubiquity of transference in human relationships. For, to desire the (powerful) other distorts the experiencing self, because the self as creating the found objective world is eclipsed. Here we can say, following Andre Green's (1975, p. 13a) lead, that there is no such thing as a patient, only a particular patient with a particular analyst. This is what Roustang means, I believe, by interplay: the two must fit and meet preconsciously their mutual needs and desires. The analyst has to be, as it were, the right kind of knowing–giving other, the patient the right kind of pained self who will learn the analyst's language, his or her speech, i.e., his or her metaphors. That the analyst structures and allows this distortion is the most minimal reading of his role in the interplay; that he does this ultimately in the service of resolving transference is one of the paradoxes of psychoanalysis.[12] Transference desire, to reiterate, creates the other as authority. Thus its inherent distortion: what was a developmental necessity (i.e., the subordination of the child to the care-taking people helping that child negotiate the various developmental stages) becomes, given environmental pathology, a neurotic (transference) problem as it aggravates narcissistic issues and fosters the anxious ego. Desire, in this perspective, becomes the basis of transference distortion. In analysis, it is the knowing other, as analyst, who interprets the subject's desire. Transference desire creates the analyst as interpreter, otherwise the subject would not come to have

10 Newtonian psychology is a term coined by Capra (1982). See his discussion of psychoanalysis (pp. 164–188).

11 For a brilliant study of transference in the analytic community, see Roustang (1982). I am singularly indebted to Roustang (1982, 1983) for stimulating my thoughts in this chapter.

12 Perhaps we metamorphose our experiences in order to hide the distortions inherent in our desires. For a perceptive study of this issue, see Romanyshyn (1983).

someone else explain the meaning of his own symptoms.[13] To use an example from the Book of Genesis, Pharaoh had Joseph interpret his dreams; by not knowing the meaning of his dreams, he blinded himself (defenses). In the process, he gave authority to Joseph, who became the knowing, powerful other. A patriarchal god gives Joseph the talent of interpreting – showing how authority perpetuates its image as the knowing other.[14]

Interplay entails polarity, and the polarity of authority entails the other as knowing and the self as unknowing, or in need of the other. Developmentally, as we have indicated, one has little choice: he or she must learn to negotiate infantile desires while experiencing maturational need for the other. The outcome of this task is crucial. When the child experiences a basic sense of equality between developmental need and gratification, he or she has the opportunity to fill in the space between the *me* and the *not me* with created/found reality. When desire arises from such developmentally relational experiences (desire as relational), authority is recognized as given but is not submitted to as the powerful or all-giving other. Where the anxious ego predominates, desire takes on the negative aspects we delineate as transference desire. Using Platonic metaphors to describe this unknowing self, the narcissistic anxious ego, we would speak of the subject lost in the darkness of forgetfulness; remembering means knowing the meaning of one's desires. But to know one's desires is to analyze them, to interpret them, i.e., again to recognize that desire subordinates the *wanting* subject to the *possessing* other, or the authority.[15]

Transference creates the analyst as analyst. Where the patient cannot initially create the analyst as analyst, there can be no resolution of desire, no resolution of transference. Termination occurs when the analyst facilitates the eventual resolution of transference desire, instead of perpetuating it. If the analyst perpetuates transference, he or she engenders, to use Ricoeur's (1970) evocative phrase, a *hidden complicity with death* inherent in the human situation. When the

---

13 See Roustang (1983), particularly Chapter 3, for a stimulating discussion elaborating on this approach.

14 Recourse to the other in the analytic tradition entails transference; recourse to the other in western religious tradition entails idolatry. One is reminded of Meister Eckhart's 'mystical atheism' as expressed in such sentiments as, 'So therefore let us pray to God that we may be free of "God"' (in McGinn, 2001, p. 145 and Colledge and McGinn, 1981, p. 200).

15 In this chapter, I am accepting the traditional western distinction between spirituality and organized religion. I return to this distinction later in my discussion of spirituality (internality), Meister Eckhart, and the experience of desire.

analyst stands over against the patient, as the powerful knowing other, he perpetuates the anxious ego and/or asks the patient to submit to ideology. Ideally both the analyst and his or her knowledge have to be learned (incorporated?) and then forgotten by the patient in order for the patient to recognize authority without submitting to it.

Roustang suggests that the need for the knowing other, particularly in psychoanalysis, comes out of our fear of personal madness and delirium, the isolation of our own associative images. From Roustang's perspective, both theory and religious dogma serve similar functions: they provide a common language as well as an objective boundary to balance the unboundedness of personal associations and fantasies. We could summarize his position by saying that the analyst's idiosyncratic matching of the patient's associations is a potential psychological moment of creativity and, simultaneously, bewilderment. Thus, Roustang speaks of the need for a common language, a theory, so that the individual is not lost in the privacy of his or her associations. The individual here means both the patient and the analyst (Roustang, 1983). Although there is great creativity in this line of thought, it does not seem to fully appreciate the structural issues behind desire and the other. As indicated above, humans are developmentally dependent on the care-taking other for survival. In the course of negotiating this enormous dependency, he or she has to face the satisfaction of infantile instinctual gratifications tied to this needed other – hence the inherent possibility (probability) of distortion in the experience of the self and the other. What we have called the anxious ego, following Fingarette (1963), seems to be of common occurrence, suggesting that the ideal fit of developmental needs, self-respect, and the maturational environment is indeed rare, at this present historical stage of child-rearing.

Eckhart alludes to internality as the other side of externality. Using Platonic metaphors, he maintains that true internal awareness (openness) is simultaneously awareness (openness) of the world (as other). Eckhart understood that the achievement of this openness was a developmental task, a positive goal for human consciousness to achieve. Freud and Winnicott speak to the same issues. In paraphrasing their thought, we would say that openness to the quiet center of the self (Winnicott) entails resolution of the narcissistic defenses (Freud), which means experiencing the capacity to make the world real by loving it. As Roustang reminds us, however, this other, this loved-world-as-other, is not the knowing powerful other (transference other), the other who judges me, the other who gives me thoughts to think, ideology to follow, or words to say. Rather, the other is simply the other, the non-transference other, the interface of my subjectivity, the relational other giving birth to what I call relational desire.

The world exists and is constantly recreated at the edge of the me and the not-me. Such internality, which Eckhart speaks of and which psychoanalysis is likewise aware of, locates the knowing other as inside the self, as well as the known-other, the world, as simultaneously internal and external. True internal awareness is awareness of the world, Eckhart concluded. Self-valuation and care for the world are equal expressions. When this occurs, transference desire is sublimated into insight. The narcissistic anxious ego has thus significantly receded. Both the insightful person, who knows the world because he or she knows him- or herself and the person who is comfortable with both personal aloneness and personal delirium replace the desiring self, the Pharaoh, who has to have his Joseph. Such a stage of development provides a person with the ability to interpose insight between desire and the other. Therefore an individual becomes capable of assuming responsibility for his or her actions because insight resolves the transference by giving back to the patient the authority he or she invested in the powerful other. What is left is only relational desire, where the polarity of subject/object has been resolved or, to view it more cautiously, significantly lessened.

Western religion, and its particular metaphors, is a clear example of the issues of authority and the self, transference and the interplay of desire. This is so because it establishes *the knowing other* as a protection against the traumas of the anxious ego, i.e., immortality against death. Dogmatism attempts to find and to bind the powerful knowing other, the truth, via a formulated theory and prescribed practice. The knowing other is found and, because of the desire to possess or control the knowing other, perception conforms. Such transference to the powerful knowing other is, however, not limited to religious organizations. It occurs whenever theory is articulated as normative rather than informative, whenever theory dictates prescribed technique rather than encouraging personal verifiability. To phrase this thought in a Winnicottian schema: it is seen whenever theory is simply found and not simultaneously created. Such is the legacy of dogmatism, which inevitably eventuates in sectarianism. Freud (1974, p. 98) was aware of the dangers of such a religious transference occurring within psychoanalysis. Note his comments to Jung:

> Transference on a religious basis would strike me as most disastrous; it could only end in apostasy, thanks to the universal human tendency to keep making new prints of the cliché's we bear within us. I shall do my best to show you that I am unfit to be an object of worship.

Analysts, given their own unrecognized transference, can likewise yearn for the powerful other who knows, and in the process forget the tasks of self-knowledge, self-centering, and self-forgetting that are a byproduct of the pursuit of truth. As transference desire is so intimately tied to the experience of the other, it becomes possible to speak about the almost universal presence of the (neuroticized) religious authority metaphor. Freud's injunction to Jung is really an injunction to the profession of psychoanalysis: avoid falling into a religious transference. Roustang (1982, p. 72), following this line of thought, notes that:

> If the analyst relies entirely on himself in practice, he cannot rely on someone else in theory. To dissociate the two makes no sense, because theorization can take place only during practice; otherwise, one will fall back either into ineffable noncommunication or into a game of love and hate, which is bound to become vicious . . .

Authority as the knowing other has to be resolved, or creativity is killed in subordination to the knowing other. To have any shibboleth in psychoanalytic theory and practice that does not include constant curiosity and questioning entails psychoanalysis acting out the religious transference. Psychoanalytic theory as a communicable, teachable science is a statement about history, about what we already know. However, as a living practice it is of necessity idiosyncratic – as idiosyncratic as the individualized smell on the transitional teddy bear, yet as common as the nose that can smell it. Theory as practice is a living bridge between patient and analyst, which the analyst and the patient construct repeatedly. The personal history of the patient (what happened) must not only be found (i.e., reconstructed), but also, in some real sense, created. Andre Green (1975, p. 12a) writes:

> In the end the real analytic object is neither on the patient's side nor on the analyst's but in the meeting of these two communications in the potential space which lies between them, limited by the setting which is broken at each separation and reconstituted at each new meeting. The analyst does

not only unveil a hidden meaning. He constructs a meaning which has never been created before the analytic relationship began.

Such an experience of the interplay of the found and the created is most difficult. It entails avoiding the isolation of personal delirium for analyst and patient, and the flight to authority, the hunger for the mother tongue that will dictate what to do and what to say. In actuality, as any practitioner knows, the analytic experience is always ambiguous to the extent that one addresses the relationship other while attempting to resolve the transference other. One either lives with this ambiguity or takes flight to the acknowledged father, the knowing other – the orthodox mandate. A common language, Roustang reminds us, is not only a way of assuring our capacity to communicate but also a net that assures us that we are held, that our *mad* personal associations are articulable. In this regard, we can note that to lessen the power of the other is to be more comfortable with personal madness – it is also to have resolved the mix-up of infantile desire and developmental need. To resolve the developmental predispositions supporting the powerful other is, as noted above, to experience the world on equal terms with the self. Internal awareness is awareness of the world.

Although insight expands the self, authority, as the knowing other, controls the self. Insight leads to the liberated consciousness that authors such as Marcuse (1955), Brown (1959, 1966), and Fingarette (1963) speak of. This is a type of consciousness where there is little or no difference between a true awareness of internality and responsiveness to the world. The world is still made real by loving it, but the division between self/object love and love for the world is seen to be illusory – the division is a product of the narcissistic anxious ego. When Erikson (1964) spoke about the goal of analysis resulting in a capacity to will the inevitable, that which has happened to us, he was speaking, I believe, about a capacity to resolve transference desire so that it conforms to fate. To do this is to be freed from the search for the all-powerful knowing other. When one is no longer subject to the transference desire, one is able to live freely and creatively in the world. Freud was not Reichian when he said the goal of analysis was to be able to love and to work; nor do I think he was, in using the word love, arguing for a delusional state. He was talking about a state of consciousness that exhibits minimal ambiguity toward that which fate has dealt us. With this comes a capacity to manifest care as discussed by Erikson, the capacity to promote and sustain a maternal good-enough environment as described by Winnicott or, finally, Eckhart's understanding of compassion for the world, free from the demands of distorting desire.

In the perpetual battle of Eros and Thanatos, psychoanalysis is a weapon for growth and unity; through it we are able to look back on ourselves, to be in wonder at the poetry that is ourselves. In healing the distortions of transference desire and in expanding the possibility of relationship desire, the process of human awareness has reached a new level of compassion and care. That Freud sparked this development leaves us forever in his debt.

SECTION 2
CLINICAL STUDIES:
IN SEARCH OF A SELF

CHAPTER 6

Language, love, and healing[1]

I would like to approach the question of healing in psychoanalysis by paraphrasing Winnicott's prayer (which by now has been over-quoted), namely that we be alive when we die. A hope that, I believe, should be an essential goal for patients as well as for analysts. Winnicott also noted that feeling alive, feeling real, could not be simply equated with the satisfaction of our instincts. He wrote that our instincts are personalized, so to speak, when they support and are in unison with our personal goals. Freud hinted at a similar process in his famous dictum that where id is, ego shall be. If to be alive is to experience oneself as real, experiencing creativity as well as personal initiative, then we have a usable context in which to understand psychoanalytic work.

Psychoanalysts and psychotherapists do not simply uncover what was buried, so to speak, although they certainly do that. They do not simply identify, confront, and interpret various developmental defenses, although they undoubtedly do that also. In this journey toward realness, toward aliveness, analysts, and therapists, try to provide a safe place where patients can find, and re-find, their personal history – a place where the language of their symptoms, of their non-aliveness, can be heard. Psychoanalysts attempt to provide a quiet place where therapeutic caring can quietly and patiently sustain a patient's grief – a caring one might legitimately speak of as love. In such a setting, the rifts within us and between us, the dividing fissures, the pathologies from narcissistic to neurotic disorders, have the possibility of coming together. Such a coming together, within oneself and with each other, is a healing worth striving for – a healing that should have as one of its

---

1 This chapter was originally presented at a conference on healing sponsored by the Council of Psychoanalytic Psychotherapists and the American Association of Pastoral Counselors in April 1999.

ingredients, for analyst and analysand, a demonstrable capacity for vulnerability, compassion, and civility, for oneself as well as for others. What I have just stated is by way of introduction to my personal reflections about psychoanalytic work – a work I have thought about, in terms of what I am doing and why I am doing it, for over 30 years.

The ancient Greeks noted that happiness – I think we can read this in the context of aliveness – resided in the full exercise of personal competence. Freud echoes this theme when he notes that the goal of analysis is to enable a person to love and to work. It is within this context that we can understand what might seem like a more pessimistic conclusion of Freud's, namely that at the end of an analysis a patient exchanges neurotic (he spoke of hysterical) 'misery for common unhappiness' (Freud, 1893–1895, p. 305). Although I have always had a sense of what Freud meant, writing this short chapter has helped me understand common unhappiness anew. Common unhappiness, I have come to appreciate, need not be experienced as a dour sadness. It has more to do with the acceptance of death, conflict, and ambiguity in the ongoing task of integrating one's personal histories. When we are able to arrive at such an emotional integration, we have the *possibility* that the rift between our unrealistic wishes and/or ideals and our historical actuality can be bridged. I believe this is what Erikson (1964) had in mind when he noted in *Insight and Responsibility* that we are most free (i.e., most alive) when we are able 'to will the inevitable' that has happened to us (p. 118). We are alive when we know both intellectually and emotionally, and have mourned for, what we have lived through. We are personally grounded to the degree that we accept the present moment and relinquish the fantasies of what we would have liked to have happened, or even, in a fairer world, what should have happened. We are alive when we can interact with those with whom we live, with those whom we love, not as salves for our injuries but as possibilities for experiences. To be able to use oneself, to be able to use one's world, not in a manipulative sense but by experiencing creative and mutual relationships, is to feel effective. Winnicott has these experiences in mind, I believe, when he speaks about being alive. Feeling alive, feeling grounded, as well as being intimately connected with others, is, however, a life task; it is not an existential given. In psychoanalysis, such a task is negotiated essentially by a therapeutic relationship, mediated through personal and interpersonal dialogue.

As patients recognize and attempt to resolve the old scripts of their lives, they can be more actively immersed in the world. As they have walked the difficult streets of their pasts, they need no longer be held, in solitary captivity, by their histories. Therapy offers the possibility of being real rather than reactive. The human condition, what I believe Freud alluded to when speaking of common unhappiness, can be accepted and lived with. Within such a context, we can speak of healing.

Walking the streets of one's past, in psychoanalytic therapy, means understanding how we have been spoken to and therefore how we speak. The words that pass between patient and analyst provide alternative readings, alternative metaphors for our desires and our loves, our experiences and our needs.

What I have indicated about healing implies, as I have stated, understanding psychoanalysis and psychotherapy metaphorically. Elaborating on these thoughts, I noted (Gargiulo, 1998a, pp. 416–417) that:

> . . . a metaphor is, as we know, that which evokes something else – a use of analogy to promote a depth of meaning and emotional resonance, as when we speak, for example, of the evening of life. Just as a metaphor points to something else, locates the center of meaning somewhere else, [it is important to] remember that ultimately there is not, nor can there be, one definitive center of meaning. By the very nature of our capacity to use metaphor, we are guaranteed continuous new meanings.
>
> What do I mean when I say that psychoanalysis is a metaphor? To speak of something as unconscious, for example, is to [place within a] context an individual's self-understanding. When we say that the unconscious is revealed or found as it is interpreted, we are describing an aspect of self-knowledge that comes in many guises. That is, knowing ourselves is also to experience not knowing ourselves, turning our eyes away from or even refusing to see ourselves. The metaphorical nature of the unconscious is equally true of such concepts as resistance, transference, idealized self-object or transitional space, *inter alia*.
>
> We can also speak of desire itself as a metaphor for the other . . . the other as culture, the other which germinates desire within us; even the prohibition of desire is the other, as superego.

When we understand transference as a metaphor, for example, we are attempting to elucidate how we are contextual creations, made up of our many histories and our many desires. We can appreciate that when patients are, for the psychological moment, their forgotten childhood dreams, fears, hopes, or expectations, they nevertheless encompass more than meets the ear, at that moment. Transference, in this context, can be understood as a metaphor for memory, for our need to speak the language spoken to us, for the ambiguity of desire and sometimes the absence of desire, as well as the different selves desires evoke. That we are all had by our histories and by what we do with those histories is not in itself a statement of pathology but of the dilemma of self-understanding. To understand the Freudian metaphors of the mind – id, ego, superego, conscious, preconscious, and unconscious – is, in fact, to appreciate man and woman as divided. To understand the metaphors of defense is to appreciate men and women as warring within themselves. Psychoanalysis offers, as far as is individually and humanly possible, a place where another will listen, with minimal judgment, to our story – a place where another will help us understand how we are telling it, point out our forgetting, our possible distortions, as well as our re-enactments. As language and emotion become safe, as memory becomes clear, as re-enactment becomes difficult, we are achieving a healing from neurotic misery to common unhappiness – a common unhappiness, I repeat, that is not a dour sadness but an acceptance of the ambiguities and conflicts of life, the reality of death, and the need to continuously examine our lives.

The recognition of common unhappiness is, as I have mentioned, no morose outcome to treatment; it is similar, I believe, to Winnicott's conviction of the universality of an everyday mild depression – a mild depression that is concomitant with the recognition of our historical place in the world, as well as the experience of our inner aloneness.

If we are listened to with compassion and respect, we should be able to find these qualities in ourselves. If we are listened to with a neutral ear, so to speak, we should find human differences more acceptable and thus be able to experience vulnerability as well as civility. Civility grows out of the awareness of the respect and care we owe others as well as ourselves. Terminating therapy, an individual should be able to love the world and to experience personal competence, to value him- or herself and be committed to the surprise of finding out who he or she is with honesty and humor. To know how and where we stand with ourselves and with others is essential to being alive. Finding oneself in the dialogues of therapy means walking a path that makes the journey out of the dark forest of our pathologies possible rather than just frightening. We know our aloneness, however, because we are with others. Paradoxically when we are not in relation with others we are not alone, we are isolated.

The experience and awareness of personal aloneness can be a contented and grounded place for many individuals. For others, seeking a spiritual interpretation of the human enterprise, it is a seedbed for understanding whatever transcendent reality may be beyond them. Whitehead (1960) concluded that 'religion is what the individual does with his own solitariness' (p. 16). If one accepts such a definition, we can see that the human issues that psychoanalysis addresses, the profound subjectivity as well as relatedness of human awareness, dovetail with many spiritual traditions. Psychoanalytic healing, in my judgment, need not pre-empt either the acceptance of the finality of our historical actuality or the possibility of a transcendent context for knowing and experiencing our humanity.

Although it is possible to argue that the most pervasive and viable *interpretation* an analyst makes to a patient is the quality of the therapeutic relationship, it is particularly important for analysts to remember that such a therapeutic relationship is a two-way street. An analyst must find healing also. Although we can presume an analyst's competence, we need not require brilliance. Although we can expect intellectual honesty, we can hope that an analyst is able to manage his or her self-referential narcissism. The intellectual and emotional milieu out of which an analyst's own healing can occur entails his or her being able to study whatever insights a psychoanalytic perspective can provide, knowing, without intellectual cynicism, that one is not able to hold truth except as a point of reference.

Healing, as I have tried to convey, is a two-edged sword: both patient and analyst are its subjects. Helping others find and own their lives can, and frequently does, awaken an analyst's own shadows; he or she comes to healing with each case he or she treats. We can speak, consequently, of the analyst's common unhappiness as found in this repetitive healing. If the two-edged sword of healing does not cut into the analyst's side, he or she will sacrifice a little bit of life, a little bit of aliveness, a little bit of realness. Consequently, for both patient and analyst, the task of finding life, of reaching each other, of touching the real, continues. It is not a task that one completes; it is simply a road one decides to take.

CHAPTER 7

Empathy and reverie

As psychoanalysts and therapists have learned to appreciate process over content, they have brought to the fore the importance of empathy in understanding and relating to another human being. Can one human being understand another? What does it mean to stand in another person's shoes? It certainly means more than having an intellectual grasp of his or her feelings, thoughts, and/or motivations. Does it have to do with being him or her, with allowing him- or herself to take on the shape of his or her inner terrain? And if we do so, does that mean that empathy enables us to walk on level ground with another? Freud understood that in order to hear another person we have to be able to hear ourselves. By extension we can say that in order to feel another person, to walk his or her path, we have to be able to feel ourselves, to have full access to the range of feelings of which we humans are capable. In the tradition of the Roman essayist and dramatist Terence, we have to be able to count *nothing human as alien*. Simple enough words, even profound, but difficult to live.

Caught in the web of the personal, historical, and cultural moments in which we live, we are molded by such forces to see and to feel the world in a particular manner. Our particular history, in all its ramifications, makes our life relative. Human history shows us, however, that we are constantly tempted to make our perceptions, our thoughts, and our values absolute – as if in doing so we are buffered against the momentary. In our anxiety to have a place to stand firmly, we often define ourselves as against, as different from the other – the other as *other* person, as *other* world, the *other's* thoughts, the *other's* feelings. If we are lucky, such defensive maneuvers prove unworkable. We need empathy as a bridge from our momentary selves, our own historical 'I', to this other world we experience. Paradoxically, however, to walk this bridge to the other we have to go back into ourselves, we have to allow ourselves to feel our pain, our joys, our triumphs, and our mishaps.

How do we do this? I am sure that there are many possible explanations. I would like to mention one possibility, namely our capacity for reverie. Reverie, although suggesting pathos, has more to do with memory mixed with a little make-believe, with desire reaching for the possible. It has been dismissed, for the most part, as not being a valid conduit of knowledge – as being subjectivity, the arena of poets. Yet reverie is much more than that; it is a bridge between listening ears. Only in listening to the echoes of our memories can we hear the depth of meaning of another's words. Our capacity for empathy and reverie and their role in helping us know each other is suggestive of the medieval philosophical inquiry as to whether there is one mind, with many manifestations, or, as would seem most obvious on first viewing, many minds. Such a question is actually not the result of ungrounded theoretical speculation but reflects a dim awareness of the universality of human consciousness – a premise psychoanalysis has operated by in its understanding of drives, defenses, and the unconscious since its inception. Freud thought that to know one mind and its conflicts was to know of human conflicts in general. (Telepathy and clairvoyance, subjects that both Sandor Ferenczi and Freud had great interest in, become more understandable within this context.)

Empathy is not extrinsic to experiencing another person; it is intrinsic. A physician without empathy is dangerous, a teacher without empathy alienating, a friend without empathy a stranger, and a psychotherapist without empathy not only ignorant but also useless. All this is rather obvious. What I would like to highlight is the role of reverie in our capacity to experience empathy in a clinical setting – a capacity close to Freud's notion of free hovering attention – a capacity that Theodor Reik (1948) likewise emphasized in his description about how we humans hear each other.

As a patient tells his or her story, we have to be writing our own autobiography. Is that, perhaps, the patient's gift to us – in order to hear them we have to re-find and re-own our lives? Age does not seem to limit the endless corners of memories, thoughts, or phantasies where we can find ourselves as we interact with others. The following case will, I hope, clarify my use of reverie and empathy in a clinical setting.

Thinking about my first few years in practice, my mind goes to a particular young man I treated. Why is it that I think of Gary? He was, as he comes back to me, a quiet man who seemed particularly out of place in the busyness of mid-Manhattan. Do I merge him with memories of myself, aged 10, who, before graduating sixth-grade grammar school, participated in a school show pantomiming a dunce to the music of *I'm Forever Blowing Bubbles*? As I remember that dark-eyed little boy responding to the audience's laughter and applause, I recall being both pleased and puzzled by my situation. I was able to play the dunce and anticipate the unexpected in this self-choreographed pantomime, all the while having such difficulty learning in the classroom.

So perhaps it was myself that was the backdrop for my memories of Gary. The image of that puzzled, isolated, young boy echoed in my mind as I encountered this lonely, pale young man. Gary, as I remember him, seemed both innocent and bewildered; he was hardly able to articulate why he was in my office at all. I felt not only concern but also protective of this stranger. I was, initially, puzzled by my feelings. He was a carpenter, as well as a political activist, i.e., he participated in Marxist study groups. He spoke of his father, who had left the family many years ago, as well as his mother in such distant terms that I was barely able to sense their presence. He grew up in a country farm environment, of Swedish ancestry, and had, just a year or so ago, moved to New York City. Tall and blond, in his early 20s, Gary was awkward in his movements. After work, except when he went to his discussion groups, he would go to his apartment and either read or play the piano. Gary had no girlfriends and showed no indications of any sexual conflicts; he seemed to be asexual and non-aggressive in his responses to others.

Gary was a likeable young man, as are most injured people who do not run away from their pain. After speaking of his personal history, he was quite content to sit opposite me, on a twice-a-week basis, and say nothing, often for 5–10 minutes, to my listening ears. If I asked a direct question, he would answer, and then very briefly.

I had been taught (during the mid-1960s) to listen carefully and consistently to patients. I had been taught that their free speech, so to speak, would lead us into forgotten terrains. I had not been taught how to respond to silent flatness. I began to feel inept and mildly irritated. To my gentle reminders that he try to say whatever might occur to him with as little self-judgment as possible, Gary would smile uncomfortably while conveying bewilderment as to how he was supposed to speak of his insides. After a few months of what seemed like a standoff, it became clear to me that I was not handling this case well. Gary wondered if therapy was for him, while I, in my beginner's enthusiasm, felt frustrated. The evocation of need was painful for me. Had not my white-haired psychiatrist from my childhood made me feel safe and understood? Had not other therapists I had seen, even before my formal analysis, been of help when I was struggling to put into words my own discontents? In view of such memories, I was unwilling to lay the absence of progress solely at the feet of my patient.

I do not remember when it occurred to me to ask the most obvious of questions; in retrospect, I am embarrassed by its simplicity. One session, I asked Gary what it was like when there was so much silence between us. And in a quiet, calm voice he said that he was used to it. There was, he continued, hardly any speaking in his household when he was growing up. At the dinner table, for example, only the most perfunctory of interchanges would occur (e.g., 'Can I have more potatoes?'). After dinner, he would go to his room, play the piano, or read. Occasionally he would hear his parents fighting. When he said this it became clear that our work together was not making headway because it was, in fact, repeating and replicating Gary's childhood experiences. That was why he did not experience my relatively silent presence as a possibility for self-discovery. Gary did not know, in practice, anything about personal communicating. The space between us was cluttered with a dead emptiness.

I recall wondering whether I had re-found George, my classmate from eighth grade. George, who would not speak to anyone when our class was in the schoolyard; George, whose face was white with fear and who seemed to hear only with his eyes. I remember walking up to him and saying that I, too, was frightened and that it was okay to talk, I would listen. George would not answer me; he would nervously smile, acknowledge my presence and then walk away. I knew that for all the difficulties I had at home, with an angry and demanding father, I had, paradoxically, with my parents' vitality, links to the world. Gary brought to mind not only my childhood but also George, imprisoned by his fears.

Fortunately I was beginning to read the works of Donald Winnicott and was gaining a familiarity with the concept of a *play-space* between patient and analyst. Gary, I began to think, could not communicate in any playful interactive way because he had been so injured by self-absorbed and remarkably non-communicative parents; his injuries were as real as if he had been physically abused.

If Gary had no bridge to reach me, then I would give him words, as building blocks. I decided, therefore, to speak and no longer to quietly wait for his associations. I spoke about anything that touched on Gary's world: carpentry, politics, piano playing, etc. Gary listened and did not turn away as George had. And ever so slowly he began to answer, not with the dead language he had used until then but, almost imperceptibly, with a growing presence of tone and color in his voice and a desire to connect in his intentions.

I had changed my approach, however, not without misgivings. I had recently left full-time college teaching with some regret; had I, perhaps, fallen back into it? Was I, in my more active responses to Gary, substituting a personal need to be the good father for an analytic discipline that would, presumptively, be a better guarantee of the patient's eventual autonomy? I read as much of Winnicott as possible, as well as Ferenczi; I knew that the words I read would not have any strength until I could make them real by my interactions with Gary. Is that what Winnicott meant by each individual's task to *create* the *found* world? But at this early stage of my analytic practice I was operating more on intuition than on intellectual conviction. Only as I experienced Gary's more personal responses were my concerns lessened.

Gary continued for another year, sitting opposite me twice weekly, before he accepted my thought that he come more frequently and try using the couch. Even when he was experiencing analysis in a more traditional way, however, I tried not to lose sight of the therapy playground in which we found ourselves. As we worked together, Gary understood how his parents' disconnected emotional relationship with him had abused him, by omission, and had left him stranded in his own inner world. As this awareness took root in him, he was, as I look back on it now, at an adolescent stage of development, figuratively speaking. This developmental stage was dramatically brought home to me when, one session, he announced that his Marxist study group had concluded that psychoanalytic therapy was oppressive and designed to support a paternalistic, capitalistic economic system. He continued, as if reciting a script, that if he continued to pay my fee, he was, in fact, supporting a system that celebrated a capitalistic reward for the performance of a necessary human task. Furthermore, he proclaimed, since he earned considerably less an hour than I did, I was, in fact, exploiting him with the arbitrary fee I had set.

I was taken aback by his statements and fell back on what I supposed were the underlying issues, at least as I had understood what I had been taught about transference. I spoke of his forgotten and repressed rage at his father, as well as his distrust of his distant mother. I tried to relate his rage at exploitation to the lack of personal care evident in his early home and to his feeling that there was no way he could affect the parental circle. All to no avail. Gary decided to leave therapy.

At this point, frustrated by my not getting anywhere, I asked if he saw any solution to the inequality he had come to articulate and to hate. He said, after some minutes of silence, that the only way he could establish equality between us was if he paid me what he himself earned, three-and-a-half dollars an hour. (Somewhere on the edge of my consciousness, I remembered working in my own father's store, feeling both exploited and powerless.) It did not take me long to agree. I wasn't sure quite what I was doing, but I knew that Gary needed to feel that the ground between us was level. I also knew that I did not want to lose Gary as a patient; we had both worked too hard to get where we were. Our financial arrangement lasted for about one and a half years.

We continued our work together, and at the end of this period of time Gary began joking with me that as his business improved he was going to charge the same outrageous fees I did. He added, around this time, that he had been thinking that, since I had mastered more than he had for now, he could pay me my fee without feeling exploited.

In retrospect, I understand that I was able to let Gary create his world via his relationship with me, rather than just interpret his need to do so. I was able to provide building-block words that helped Gary articulate his feelings, particularly those of exploitation and oppression. By agreeing to a change in fee, I gave him power over my income. As I look back, after so many years, I am convinced that my personal reveries enabled me to hear Gary's yearning to connect. As my mind wandered among the memories, as well as the pain, of my own exploitative father, because my reveries slipped back to the school yard of P.S. 68 in the northeast Bronx and to my friend George, who never spoke back to me, because my own distracted mother had, at least, kept talking to me and because the psychiatrist during my tenth year of life had been so considerate – for these, and other reasons, I could be Gary's other side – the side facing the world, the side he needed if he would ever be able to re-find his own childhood and have some mastery over its events.

Gary stayed another 2 years or so and left feeling more alive, less frightened, and in better command of himself. A year before he left, however, he said, rather blandly one day, that his mother had called and told him that the father he had not seen for years had collapsed in a small southern fishing village, the victim of a sudden heart attack. Although I spoke about his feelings for his lost, now dead, father, I was not able to relieve the range of anger, as well as grief, I suspected was there.

I had been the good environment Gary needed – perhaps too much so. I still had a great deal to learn about the analytic playground. Notwithstanding all of our work together, Gary left treatment, I believe, somewhat prematurely. He was, however, anxious to be out on his own, and he did not think we could go much further. I agreed, because whatever reservations I had were overshadowed by his desire and his capacity to take fuller ownership of his life. He left, as I have said, a happier, warm young man. There were smiles where only bewilderment had been, color where before I had seen only pallor, personal ambition instead of isolating depression. He was living with a girlfriend at the time; the relationship was serious and satisfying. He called a number of months after he left, to tell me that he was getting married. I have not heard from him since.

If I think about empathy, I suppose I would characterize it as a willingness to symbolically revisit the wounding experiences of our own lives in order to find common ground with another. My own reverie, revisiting some of my childhood experiences, enabled me to find such a space where both Gary and I could walk.

Gary is part of my memories and my reveries and so I am still walking with him while I listen to others tell their tales. I know now that Gary helped me find myself as a psychoanalyst. As the years gather in his life, I hope Gary will be able to muse and revisit not only his therapy but also what was good in his childhood. In doing so, he will find himself once more.

CHAPTER 8

Reflections, musings, and interventions: a personal communication on psychoanalytic work

Reflections

I have often thought that our lives are a little more than a gathering of days, our childhood lost to both memory and forgetting; for the rest, we scramble to make sense of what happens to us. As a psychoanalyst, I have spent my days pondering what it is I do as well as what is done to me. Do my patients affect me by expecting me to be somehow above it all, to be knowing and insightful, compassionate yet strong, intelligent and yet unchallenging to their lifestyles? For the most part, I respond as best I can. But I owe it to myself as well as to my patients to ask if my response is real or if it is a false self, a professional persona I become in order to be known in some knowable way. Who teaches us the ways to be known? Parents, teachers, colleagues, and patients – the *other* in human experience. Include as well a society that has fulfilled Freud's dire prediction: America, he mused, will make psychoanalysis a private business.

Indeed. A private business with all the need to supply a capitalist rationale: a product, self-understanding, and/or adaptability. Something I can sell to *them*. My patients are, for the most part, 25 to 60 years old who come to me hoping that I can do something for them, and they will be happier or less sad, less anxious, or less likely to fall off the cliff we all walk along, but few are able to acknowledge.

Through all this, a question persists: did I go into this profession to free myself or to help others? Is there a difference?

While I am working with someone, I cannot take notes. I do not believe it useful to try to keep track, particularly in a cognitive sense, of what's going on in a therapeutic experience. For me, writing either during or immediately after the session, or continually evaluating diagnosis and/or prognosis, is a subtle intrusion into experiencing the

69

patient. (In fact, I get easily distracted when I read case presentations in which there are predictable responses. They do not seem like anything I do.) I remember names and events, dreams, and major turning points. For the rest I listen to the patient as carefully and attentively as I am able to. I automatically think in terms of psychoanalytic categories because that is what I have been taught to think in. The psychoanalytic model is useful; I do not think it is the only approach to the psyche, but it is a way of thinking that has helped me in my own personal analysis, and so I organize what is happening with a patient in terms of childhood experiences, defenses, transference reactions, and levels of insight. Beyond these formulas, of course, I care for my patients, want to help them, as well as want to experience myself being effective. Winnicott (1958) writes about the feeling of hating a patient in his article 'Hate in the counter-transference' – knowing it and not acting on it: knowing it so that you can find its roots, in either oneself or the patient, and in the knowing and in the naming to free oneself of the burden that rage and hate bring. If such emotions are weighing a patient down in his or her sessions, if they are weighing me down in the treatment, then I know that they are weighing them down in their life outside of this cell we call a psychoanalyst's office. I live in a secular monk's room where two people dwell, for a gathering of sessions, where one meditates not on a future heaven but on a burdened now and, frequently, on a past hell. Fortunately my present office is bright, looks out over a busy street in front and a 100-year-old church to the right, with its frequent bell tolling marking the passing of light.

Musings

The case I would like to talk about, the fragments of which I remember, is one such example of a hell in the past and a burdened present. The treatment has gone on for over 12 years; we are, I believe, close to the end. The incidents I mention have occurred within the last 6 months. They have come about, I am sure, through expectable maturational growth and our analytic work together. I give some history of the patient, recall some interventions I made as well as those that the patient made, all in the hope of giving some glimpse into the way human beings have of interacting, i.e., of talking to each other. As I have mentioned, I have had a strong desire to understand this talking cure, these words that carry love and hate, understanding, and ignorance in their shapes. Maybe because of this fascination with words and how we are had by language, and how we know ourselves by language, I read poetry by all kinds of poets. Perhaps it was the poetry of Freud's writing, even in translation, that initially captivated me. Certainly it was the poetry of Winnicott's writings that led me to read more and more of him and to listen and name clinical experiences in ways that echoed him. That I have been reading him for over 30 years must surely affect my work. And, before Winnicott and Freud, I was fascinated by western philosophy, which was my major in college, and by western theology and religious studies, which comprised my master's studies. I read Freud at 15, St Thomas Aquinas at 22, and, by 30, I was reading and studying Freud again.

Psychoanalysts are not arcane gurus of the mind pronouncing, with solemnity, what is hidden in the human psyche. We are all formed by our childhoods, informed by our teachers, and instructed by our readings. If another wishes to share some of our musings, it helps to know some of the sources that have informed those musings. Along with Freud, the authors I remember with the most excitement were Groddeck and Ferenczi, Balint as well as Erikson, Theodor Reik, and, of course, Winnicott. Some I particularly respect are Otto Fenichel, Paul Ricoeur, Joseph Campbell, as well as Meister Eckhart, Francois Roustang, and Lewis Thomas. Winnicott speaks of the need for a patient to be able to play, not the play of games, but the play of interaction. Winnicott also speaks of how even the most correct interpretation has its own moment of birth in the treatment, and should not be prematurely delivered by the analyst – a lesson I learned, many times over, with this case. Roustang helped me understand that one can never teach another what words to say, or what thoughts to think; there are no words to say unless one wishes to indulge in religious rituals. Therefore, in the following account I consider it a success if I convey to the reader the kind of treatment playground that I try to foster.

Before discussing the case in any detail, I would like to share one further observation about my way of working within the therapeutic experience. Although I recognize transference as a most powerful phenomenon, I am simultaneously very suspicious of it. By that I mean that I believe an analyst should be maximally aware of what he or she brings to the relationship, before judging whether a particular patient's response or reaction is a manifestation of a distortion of the present, in view of the past. In addition I am extremely wary of what is known as an idealized transference. I not only do not encourage it, I suspect I discourage it by dropping little facts about myself and my human foibles, in order to keep the relationship precisely that – a relationship. Notwithstanding this, patients will do with this information what they will. I feel better for conducting an analysis within this style of communication. If patients have a need to distort or skew their experience of me, they will. The stance that the more neutralized the analyst is, the more antiseptic his or her responses to the patient, the clearer the transference will be, is, I believe, simply wrong. As I see it, such a stance, away from the natural personality of the analyst, clouds the transference. Michael Balint is explicit in this line of thinking; Winnicott is less explicit, although I am convinced that he clearly practiced this way. Only a completely relaxed, comfortable analyst would have thought up his famous squiggle game to begin with.

Whether I did psychoanalysis or psychotherapy with this patient, each reader will decide. I find the distinction, when asked by analysts of other analysts, to frequently reflect a religious test as to orthodoxy rather than to functioning. In this vein, I am reminded of Winnicott's response when he was asked what psychoanalysis consisted of. His answer was that that depends on who is doing it.

Interventions

The patient I would like to discuss is presently 44 years old. I have seen him, on average, twice a week for approximately 12 years. For the past 2 years I have seen him once a week with a short 15- to 20-minute telephone session spaced a few days after our meeting. (Two years ago, I moved my office from New York City to a suburb, which lengthened the trip for some patients.) It is most difficult, as I mentioned above, to encapsulate 12 years of work. I can say that the patient would, in all likelihood, be classified, when I first saw him, as schizoid with an infantile personality. Although he had a graduate degree, he was totally unfocused in his work as well as in his personal relationships. He seemed bewildered by life and by life experiences.

In therapy, the patient's life story unfolds as the work progresses. Therefore, the history I relate was gathered over a period of years and is an amalgam of the patient's words as well as analytic reconstruction. The patient grew up in an apartment in a large Midwestern city, of Jewish parents; he has one older sister.

The patient spoke of his mother as continually doting on him, the experiences of which he recognized as being destructive. She would, for example, have a potty for him when he was 10 years of age, so that if he had to urinate at night he would not have to leave the bed. Furthermore she would heat his orange juice in the morning, lest it be too cold. She was a paranoid woman who, although she worked in a position where she dealt with people daily, was totally alienated from her extensive family. As my patient was growing up, his mother frequently asked him to unsnap her bras or help her zip up her dress. She was excessively nervous whenever he crossed the street and would frequently, over his objections, want to go to his elementary school to fight his fights for him with other students. The one time she did this caused enormous humiliation for him. The patient recounted how he would wet the bed consistently until he was in early puberty. (Occasionally, during adulthood and treatment, he had short periods of wetting the bed again.)

Of his father, he hardly spoke at all. The one consistent memory was of his going on a visit with his father to relatives and returning home on the elevated train, whereupon his father got into the train a few cars ahead of his son, with no apparent thought as to whether or not his son got on the train. The patient, aged 8, walked through the train looking for his father and, when he found him, got no explanation from him as to his actions. This pattern of little or no response from his father was, in fact, a constant theme. My understanding of the father was of a severely withdrawn and depressed man, totally subordinate to his wife. (During most of the treatment, I found it difficult to remember his occupation.) The patient recalled an earlier experience when he, 4 or 5 years old, and in the midst of having a fight with his older sister, proceeded to hit her with a baseball bat. The physical damage seems to have been minimal; his parents' response was to give him a mild rebuke. A good deal of analytic clarification was necessary, however, before the patient realized the damage such permissiveness and non-paternal involvement caused.

Throughout our work, I spoke of the oedipally seductive behavior of his mother – the overdetermined, sexual, and aggressive meanings to his bed wetting, and of the rage and desolation he must have felt at being abandoned by his father. This abandonment left him bereft of a masculine image, but also left him to his sexually seductive mother. The patient recalled, frequently, that when speaking with his mother he was constantly admonished not to trust anyone, even family – that the only thing that mattered was money and that people really did not have any feelings for each other. Although making a lot of money was stressed, he was also urged to get a civil service job so that he would be secure. Furthermore, he was admonished that he should marry only a Jewish girl, because non-Jewish people were untrustworthy and frequently meant harm. (The patient had come to see me after being with a Jewish woman analyst for approximately 5 years. I have never been able to satisfactorily evaluate that work except to feel that it was not harmful in any way. Was his subsequent choice of me a move away from his paranoid mother's world?)

Reik once remarked that he did not understand analysts who spoke of liking their patients initially; he found that he was more prone to like a patient near the end of treatment rather than the beginning. This was certainly true in this case for me. It took a number of years for me to feel connected to someone whose affect was initially flat, who had childish demands on the world around him, and who used, extensively, concrete language. Although the flatness of the patient's communications caused me concern, confusion, and frequently boredom, we would work on issues centering on his infantile mode of response to his jobs, his bosses and/or fellow workers, and his occasional love relationships. Flatness is a difficult experience to convey. Although the patient was bright, I came to feel that a part of me had to be kept in hibernation, so to speak. If I interacted with what seemed to me an appropriate therapeutic pace, I was clearly beyond the patient's ability to hear and integrate. Repeatedly, therefore, I would have to remind myself and discipline myself to go slower. Throughout our work, the patient had a number of work positions and, although he whined and was demanding, he, nevertheless, had some inkling that he was not really involved effectively in the world.

For many years, the only way he spoke to this issue of effective involvement in the world was to be jealous and angry with me. These feelings showed themselves as he would continually be jealous of the money I made, the position I had, the house I had, the family I had, the car I had, and on and on. With paranoid accuracy he had guessed both the number and gender of my children and their approximate ages. When he did this, my response was merely to confirm his guess and to go on to his reactions to my family constellation. He would stay with his reaction for a few moments before going back to his conviction that, if I had anything, which he wanted, or, if other people had what he wanted, they and I were taking it away from him. This was such an emotional conviction for him that any intellectual awareness he had of its falseness was meaningless. On one occasion he accidentally met, for a few moments, both my wife and I as we were visiting the Metropolitan Museum of Art. In the next session, he offered not only a rather perceptive analysis of her manner but of her age and occupation as well.

My own musings as to how he was able to do this centered around his not being allowed to separate from his mother, at how he had been symbiotically fused to her, excited and frightened by her all at the same time, and, consequently, how these factors had delayed the closure, to use Freud's term, of his unconscious. Freud speaks of such a closure occurring around puberty; in my patient's case this was greatly delayed. I think it was this factor that enabled him to have an uncanny ability to read other people. Predictably, as he became more operationally productive in the world of work and relationships, this ability receded.

As I write this, I am also aware that, intermingled with my, at times, premature interpretations about his oedipal phantasies and realities, it was important for me to be somewhat unknowing. When I work with a patient who is overly concrete and symbiotic, it is usually helpful not to be the powerful mother/father/world, because my knowledge, or presumed knowledge, can easily intimidate the patient into complying with my interpretations or, worse, be experienced as a narcissistic injury. If I know too much, I not only know parts of them that cannot be known but in the knowing I can be experienced as transgressing upon an internal haven – that area where we are alone with ourselves, an aloneness, which Winnicott reminds us, must never be violated. When I realized that my oedipal and pre-oedipal interpretations about his anger at his father or confusion as to his boundaries were essentially getting nowhere, I simply dropped them. We worked, as indicated above, on everyday issues, of which there seemed to be an endless supply. I conveyed to the patient the realization that, if we continued to work together, he would have to help me help him, if he would ever get to where he wanted, i.e., to feel real and effective in the world and be able to love someone.

About the eighth or ninth year of our work together the patient began asking me for some books to read that might help him understand the psyche in general, as well as himself. He spoke of the numerous self-help books he was reading and asked me what I thought of them. For the most part, I did not know the specific works but I encouraged him to read whatever gave him any further sense of self-understanding. (A few of them, which I did know, I did comment on.) In addition, I mentioned some works by Winnicott and Melanie Klein, authors he was familiar with as a good friend of his was in the analytic world. Ordinarily, if there is an ordinarily in working with patients, I would discourage the intellectualization that such an approach could cause. In this case, however, I felt that the patient needed a good deal of strengthening of his intellectual grasp of human development in order to handle the primitiveness of his emotional development. It is also possible that during this time, which lasted for 2 years or so, I was exhausted and frustrated at the patient's slow progress and wanted to bring in some co-therapists to help with the treatment. I had had to come to terms, not only in this case but also in others, with the reality that some analyses would go on considerably longer than my own and that this was not necessarily a statement about my ineptitude.

I would, on occasion, find myself quite angry with both his mother and his father (anger is probably too mild a word). They had left me (they resided in Florida) with an angry, jealous, paranoid, bright, and injured child, and I was somehow supposed to bring him back to a normal life. Both mother and father were hardly *good enough* to use Winnicott's term. My frustrations were only slowly worked through as I experienced the patient's utter commitment to therapy, to work through the ghosts that haunted him, and the gates that blocked his entry into the mature world. Somewhere in the back of my mind I remembered that the patient's maternal grandfather had, at age 50, become a lawyer, after many years in a blue-collar job. This fact, which would prove a most helpful model for my patient, was, for whatever reason, blocked from my awareness until a crisis that occurred during the summer of his eleventh year of treatment.

By the time I went on my 3-week August vacation, at the end of his eleventh year, I felt that the treatment had progressed well. The over-ly concrete language had lessened, i.e., there was more emotional vitality in his speech and in our communications. The patient was set-tled into a good-paying civil service job. (Until he had more emotional flexibility, this was actually a good choice, despite mother's shadow.) He was simultaneously preparing for an alternative career. We had spent much time working on his personal relationships, and he had, as of 2 years ago, married. The marriage was a happy and satisfying one; his wife was pregnant with a much-wanted child. The jealousy and rage at me seemed to be somewhat lessened, to my relief, although I was puzzled as to how this would finally be resolved.

On my second week of vacation I got an urgent call from the patient. When I returned his call, I was met with a thoroughly enraged person who informed me that he would be stopping treatment because he had failed to get the raise he was expecting at work and another worker had gotten the position he wanted. I conveyed to him my appreciation of how upset he must feel and that it would be helpful for him to give himself a few more sessions before deciding that treatment was to be stopped. Although he agreed to this, two lengthier phone sessions, during the remaining weeks of my vacation, were necessary, because the patient was convinced that I had personally let him down with this turn of events. The intensity of the patient's regression surprised me, and I reluctantly knew that a new struggle was awaiting us. It was as if the paranoid, enraged mother had taken over and pushed aside all the work we had done. When I returned in September, I was met with a sullen, enraged but somewhat receptive patient. Somewhat receptive meant that for about 10 minutes of each session he would allow me to show him that I understood his rage, but that it had little to do with therapy, his job, or me. I mentioned that ultimately he could spend the rest of his life reactivating his mother inside him, or he could recognize that the world is not a hostile place. It (the world) is, I said, merely indifferent. To personalize it with his hate was his doing. This statement of the world as indifferent to him seemed to capture his imagination, and he would repeatedly come back to it as he began to neutralize his experiences of disappointment. (During the beginning of this turbulent time, the patient had mentioned that he wanted me to refer him to whoever had been my analyst. My response was that he wanted his grandfather back.) Each morning, for a period of about 6 to 8 weeks, I received an angry sullen message on my tape machine to the effect that he was going to quit and never come again, or that he was so depressed that he had to speak to me. When I would speak with him, for a few minutes, he would either go into rages at the unfairness of his life and the treatment he got from his parents, or he would rage at me saying that I must hate him and that I should stop it. I would quietly assure him that I felt for his anguish, and that I did not hate him. I spoke to the fact that the people he felt hate from were his manipulative, seductive mother and distant father.

After about 8 weeks of my interpretations (which had all been said many times before) and offering as much understanding as I was capable of, the patient began to repeat back to me, as if for the first time, and with a sense of personal ownership, many of the themes the treatment had touched upon. Eventually he was able to hear that he had been beating me up with his reactions and phone calls, similar to what he must have felt growing up, when his mother would never let him be. As he was able to internalize this awareness, I mentioned that I did not enjoy being beat up and that he would have to find other ways of handling his frustrations. I said this not only for self-evident reasons but because I felt (for the first time?) that the patient, as he was emerging from this dark angry place, was able to cross-identify with me, that he could experience what was happening to me and not just to himself. He was able to understand that, in making me the bad world, he was cutting off any chance of living happily. The patient was (finally?) able to experience the hatred he had inside himself for the world as other; he saw his imitation of his mother's attitudes, and began to appreciate the fact that there were objective reasons why his colleague was given the advancement, which had little to do with himself. Progressively he understood that his rage would just perpetuate his feeling injured, that it was a way of not dealing with the world, similar to the way his parents did not deal with the world.

I was fortunate enough to say two particularly helpful things during this period. One was to ask him why he kept ignoring his grandfather whom he knew well, who lived well into his 90s, and who, in the middle of his life, changed careers and fulfilled his dream of becoming a lawyer. Perhaps the patient's clue to me about wanting to see my analyst was a signal that he would be able to hear and be able to use this reference to his grandfather. The patient took to my statements with a sense of bewildered enlightenment and brought in many stories of his grandfather, showing his admiration of him and his desire to imitate his mastery of life.

My second intervention, which proved useful, was to say that he owed me some reparation for the years of jealousy and anger and for these last few months of hate. I would not accept any presents, which at first he thought I meant. I clarified that one cannot just throw people away without making reparation. I said this because I was trying to show him, I hope in not too heavy-handedly a manner, that it is possible to show concern for another, and that concern could channel productively the guilt feelings over the rage and hate that had been expressed. With this statement, he seemed to understand that he had to find and remember me as the good world, if he ever hoped to live in the good world. His manner gradually lightened, he began to joke with me much more, and he gave himself interpretations, as I mentioned above, about his previous schizophrenic type of thinking, his symbiotic as well as his oedipal tie to his mother, and his rage, now significantly modified, at his father. He continued advancing in his new business venture and began to muse about moving back to his city of birth because his new business, in the computer field, would allow him to do that. He joked that now that he was about to be a father he would have to take care of and actually think about someone else.

In the course of a few months after this crisis, he grew a beard and began to sound more mature, i.e., his voice developed a deeper resonance. His childish stance toward the world was changed and so, therefore, his physical demeanor actually matured. He let the realities of life register on him. During this period, he was diagnosed with muscular dystrophy, a mild case, but troubling nevertheless. He addressed this turn of events straightforwardly, read a great deal about his illness, joined a self-help group, and committed himself to a strict diet, to acupuncture, and to herbal supplements – all of which have proved to be very beneficial.

Epilogue

Although the case will go on for a while, I think we have passed through the eye of the storm. The sessions feel more real, the patient feels more real. Rage and hate of this particular variety, however, run deep. The solution, if one can use such a simplistic formulation, will be his achieving and sustaining a capacity for reparation and a capacity for concern. I believe his child will help him greatly in this regard. At present, I feel empathy for him with many positive feelings. I frequently find myself imagining his leaving and living a productive life.

I will be 12 or 15 years older when our gathering of days will come to an end; he will be freer and more loving, more able to use the world. I will be wiser, if a little more tired, for having worked with him. And after a while, if things go well, I will not only appreciate, further, the positive things that happened but the mistakes I made and how they fit into the treatment. In fact, the decisive move away from paranoid rage and righteousness is, I believe, a patient's willingness and capacity to use and allow for our errors, rather than vengefully retaliating for our mishaps. That this patient stayed in treatment and worked so hard is the best promise that our work will have some positive and lasting meaning.

Postscript

I have rarely written case reports; I have been greatly concerned, so I told myself, with the issue of confidentiality. I am convinced, in addition, of the impossibility of the task. Are we reporting a case's progress or creating a novelette? Secondary revision, as any clinician knows, is not limited to dream work. Having completed this case summary, I was extremely wary of reading it to the patient. I had, in the present case, less concern about the issue of confidentiality because I believed I had disguised the material sufficiently; I was wary as to what such a reading might do to the work in progress and to any possible re-enactment, in the treatment, of his sense of specialness. I attempted to handle this concern by asking a few respected colleagues what they thought my obligations were, i.e., given the particular perspective of this article, was the patient's permission a necessity and/or how would the patient experience my reading the article to him? A majority seemed to think it ethically necessary for me to get his permission; some thought it unwise for me to read the case. My concerns, nevertheless, were not lessened.

Obviously, and as was soon confirmed, something else was going on. This became clear during one session when I, unable to resolve my ambivalence, decided to read the material to the patient. What became transparent was that my concerns over the patient's experience of specialness were not validated; my feeling of loss over separation, however, was. I realized this when the patient, upon hearing the case, was quite moved and said that he felt held by me during the reading. He was, he continued, aware that our final working-together time had arrived and that my summarizing the treatment was the beginning of closure. He knew that he would miss me and, with some unbelief, that I would miss him. He spoke of being able to experience personal relationships as real, and this was clearly opening up a whole new life for him. He understood that I had not ignored him, had not walked away without a backward glance, as well as the fact that our common goal was for him to feel real and to live his own life.

We continued to work together for another year and a half, mostly on a once-a-week basis. His marriage is a deeply satisfying one but has been overshadowed by his wife's breast cancer, a cancer that they have addressed without self-pity, with courage, and with constant care for their child. He calls me every few months to let me know the state of his wife's health, as well as his own. My admiration for both of them only increases.

CHAPTER 9

Anna O.: an English object relations approach[1]

If Anna O.'s concerned mother and ailing father called upon an analyst today, what would take place? The analyst, undoubtedly, would respond by asking the parents to bring the distraught young woman into the office on a certain date, for a certain period of time, and for a stated fee. The patient would see other patients in the waiting room (the analyst would not go to her home); she would note the relative impersonality of the analyst's office, and someone who evidenced, in his or her tone of voice, no signs of parental anxiety or possible annoyance at Anna's symptoms would address her. All of this is quite obvious to us, the inheritors of Freud's legacy, but in its very commonality it contributes to a particular setting that would match the *private theater* in Anna O.'s internal world, with a distinctive therapeutic theater outside her. The analyst, in all likelihood, would respond to the patient's dramatic communications (hysterical symptoms) by seeing her as frequently as feasible; no medication would be prescribed.

The analyst would have to know internally, however, whether the seemingly psychotic symptoms were something he or she could comfortably allow to unfold or whether he or she would have to rush to understand and resolve them as soon as possible. Only if the analyst were comfortable with the primitively symbolic non-rational elements inside him- or herself could he or she allow the play to go on in a way that might allow its successful finale. Such an approach is particularly congenial to analysts who follow an English object relations model.

It is a truism that, without the living patient before one, without the personal presence, the movement of the eyes, the tone of the voice and the carriage of the body, it is difficult to have the emotional

1 This is a slightly revised version of a chapter that was published in 1984 (Gargiulo, 1984).

confirmation integral to an analysis. It is not merely metaphor that led Freud (1901–1905) to observe that the unconscious spills out from 'every pore of the body' (pp. 77–78). The historical information about Anna O., as is well known, is truncated, and, although Jones (1953), Ellenberger (1970), and Pollock (1968) have augmented our knowledge, we are essentially dealing with a literary work filtered through Breuer's defense structure. Even with all these caveats, however, the case is worth discussing. Clearly no attempt is being made to offer an empirically verifiable hypothesis; actually none need be made. Interpretations that offer a patient new, personalized internal meanings with a consequent new mode of experiencing the self are worthwhile. The value of a psychoanalytic historical reconstruction is not in its exact verifiability, or its intellectual correctness, as obviously important as these considerations are. From an object relations standpoint, the primary issue is the subjective (personal aliveness) as well as the objective (usable externality, play, and work) experience of reality that a particular line of interpretation and/or therapeutic interaction makes possible.

Before discussing the case in any detail, I would like to elaborate on these thoughts and give a very brief summary of what has come to be known as the English object relations school.

Major English authors who have written in this area, within the Freudian tradition, include Fairbairn (1954), Balint (1979), Winnicott (1958, 1965, 1971), Guntrip (1973), and Khan (1974). Such writers as these have worked with patients who are at a pre-oedipal level of personal development. Freud's theory of neurosis, with its oedipal conflict core, presupposes the existence of a person capable of using adult language and of experiencing interpersonal and therefore psychological conflict. Freud's theory of the mind and his consequent technique follow from such metapsychological presumptions. Classical technique suggests a one-person psychology, namely the patient within the treatment. Even when such pre-oedipal stages as oral, anal, and phallic are spoken of, these are approached through the oedipal model of personal emotional existence, articulated by the patient's language manifesting his or her conflict. The emphasis, again, is on the individual's pathology. The English school, on the other hand, has focused on those emotional and developmental issues that go into the making of a person. They have worked with patients whose use of language does not have the same emotional import and meaning as that of neurotically conflicted individuals – patients who feel empty or dead, or who do not (emotionally) experience that they have an inside. And using such terms as 'schizoid problems' (Guntrip), 'basic fault' (Balint), and 'true self–false self' (Winnicott) they have attempted to understand the developmental issues that give birth to the psychological person.

Within the actual treatment setting, the technical approach of this school reflects an appreciation of the role of the analyst as a contributing factor in the patient's developmental maturation, reflecting sensitivity to the mode of object relatedness that emerges in the treatment. Such an approach to patients precedes any understanding of the patient in terms of instinctual unconscious conflicts and their consequent resolution through verbal interpretation. Believing that individuals come to experience themselves as real through progressively relating to other individuals and not primarily through instinctual expression, the English school has charted areas of the mind not available to a more classical practitioner.[2] The type of patient and the issues addressed in classical therapy with neurotics are radically different from those having to do with healing a most basic split in the psyche.

From another perspective we might note the difference of approach by saying that in classical psychoanalytic treatment the area of the patient's regression is handled very cautiously and is understood frequently as a defense, as a resistance, and potentially, if not actually, as pathogenic. The patient's regression as a positive contribution to the therapeutic process is rarely spoken of. In the object relations school, on the other hand, regression, in all its forms, is spoken of and used much more extensively, with particular emphasis on the analyst's role and use of regression.

Now we can return to the patient, Anna O., to see where our line of inquiry might take us. Given the severity of her symptomatology – difficulty in speaking in coherent syntax, numerous physical conversion symptoms, extreme difficulty with vision – one could understand her parents' alarm. Furthermore, the apparent splitting of her social response into a good self and a bad self, more like a three-and-a-half-year-old naughty child, must have been puzzling and extremely disconcerting to this well-to-do, middle-class Viennese family. Her alternating selves had been obvious to the patient, and she complained of going mad. The family, probably out of a mixture of anxiety

---

2 It is the emotionally cohesive person who experiences instinctual drives as personal, otherwise they are experienced as external persecutory impingements.

and ignorance, assured her that she was not. Her moods, we are told, changed rapidly; she would hallucinate black snakes which were her hair, fingers, and various ribbons, yet she would catch herself and attempt to reassure herself of the objective reality of the world around her. Furthermore, as Breuer wrote:

> At moments when her mind was quite clear she would complain of the profound darkness in her head, of not being able to think, of becoming blind and deaf, of [as mentioned above] having two selves, a real one and an evil one which forced her to behave badly, and so on.

> Breuer and Freud (1893–1895, p. 24)

Anna had a brother younger by one year and an older sister who died at the age of 17 when Anna was 8 years old. Actually, she had had two older sisters, the first of whom died even before Anna was born. She related all of the family history, Breuer indicates, in a manner that showed her educated concern and a clear intelligence. She spoke of her extreme concern for her father, who seemed gravely ill; she spoke of how she had gotten worse herself through taking care of him; she made passing, almost casual, reference to her brother; of her mother, she spoke not at all.

Today, of course, as we have been so formed by Freud's theories, it is difficult to imagine Anna, as the daughter of an educated, wealthy Jewish family, living in a cosmopolitan center, expressing such oedipal metaphors in such an obvious way. Such issues would be addressed, of course, but within the broader context now available to us.

For the first few sessions, at least, our *literary* Anna would sit opposite me; I would not ask her to use the couch, initially, because I would want to retain eye contact with her. I would want Anna to see me until I was sure that she could use not seeing me as a way of understanding herself and not as a way of collapsing into herself. There is a difference, as Winnicott (1958) makes particularly clear, between a patient experiencing regression in the sessions (which is a goal) and withdrawal (which is an unproductive process).

In addition to the description of the symptoms above, particularly Anna's inner darkness, we can take Breuer's remarks (Breuer and Freud, 1893–1895, p. 24) as a further summary of the presenting symptoms:

> In one of these states she recognized her surroundings; she was melancholy and anxious, but relatively normal. In the other state she hallucinated and was 'naughty' – that is to say, she was abusive, used to throw cushions at

people, so far as the contractures at various times allowed, tore buttons off her bed clothes and linen with those fingers which she could move, and so on. At this stage of her illness if something had been moved in the room or someone had entered or left it (during her other state of consciousness) she would complain of having lost some time and would remark upon the gap in her train of conscious thoughts. Since those about her tried to deny this and to soothe her when she complained that she was going mad, she would, after throwing the pillows about, accuse people of doing things to her and leaving her in a muddle, etc.

In speaking with Anna, I would attempt to convey, more by tone than by verbal content, that I was not interested in finding out something about her. I would question her as to her experiences of herself during her daytime and night-time daily activities, i.e., I would not respond to her as an oddity to be cured but in fact would take her statements at face value and try to see if they had any additional meanings which could help her understand herself in a wider framework than that which had been, so far, available. I would go on to tell Anna that I understood why she spoke of herself as going mad, because her external behavior was evidencing a splitting of which she was aware. The only thing that would be questioned would be the 'tense' of her statements, i.e., that she was going mad. I would mention that she was, with this fear, remembering having gone mad, i.e., remembering a break in her sense of her own continuity of being, which occurred in her earliest childhood. Such a break, in the sense of who one is, is what we frequently refer to as *going mad.* Given Anna's subsequent development, her education, her mastery of languages, I would postulate that the (maddening) early events had happened and that she recovered, but that the recovery did not satisfactorily heal the initial break. Her reactions to her father's severe illness and her hallucinations all pointed to a disruption in the knitting together of her inner world and her interaction with the external world.

I would watch her physical reactions to our sessions very carefully, judging whether our interactions had any calming effect on the flamboyance of her symptoms. Was she able to focus her eyes in a more centered manner, for example? Were my remarks making some sense out of an inner experience of chaos, by enabling her to have the conviction that she was understood? Or, on the other hand, were my remarks possibly being experienced as intrusive, thus fostering more anxiety, with a consequent failure of the patient to be self-observing? If she were not able to use what I said, I would say to her that there was

a great deal happening to her, that we could try to understand together what may have caused her present condition, and that anything I
said was tentative. I would convey all of this in a simple, direct manner of speech.

If, on the other hand, there was more of a capacity to look at herself, which I suspect would be the case with Anna O., I would then go
on to a second major motif, namely that her conduct betrayed, and her
sense of self indicated, that she was a *bad* self and a *good* self (Anna's
words). After asking her (over many sessions) for her associative musings on what she meant by these words, I would respond by speaking
about her split experience of herself. I would be aware that we would
be dealing with an issue that Winnicott speaks of as a loss of personal
continuity of being, occurring anywhere from 18 months to 48 months
of age. I would convey to Anna that such splitting arises from conflicts
having to do with love and hate, with using and being used. Winnicott
(1971) postulates that a child goes from *relating* to an object out of
need to *using* an object, which is the emotional acknowledgment of
separation. Using an object entails mastery of aggression in terms of
negotiating effectively with the outside world. Balint (1979) speaks of
the same developmental process when he speaks of the child's *work
of conquest* vis-à-vis the important people in his emotional world.[3] The
progressive achievement of personalization, which such a *work of conquest* implies, precludes the excessive splitting that Anna manifested.

After a relatively short period of time, having had her speak about
what was going on at home and after judging, as noted above, the
effect of my words on her, I would ask Anna to use the couch. I would
see her a minimum of three times a week and, depending on her
capacity to use these sessions, would eventually increase these to four
sessions a week. I would answer most of her initial questions unless I
sensed an oedipally inquisitive or narcissistically demanding question,
in which case I would simply ask what she thought might be behind
such questions. Other questions, as general as this seems, would be
responded to, i.e., if the question applied to her. If they applied to me,
I might give some personal information, but not intimate information.
If my initial diagnosis were correct, I would be addressing a sense of

---

3 Balint goes on to state that, in his judgment, Anna O. was a case evidencing a malignant regression (in contradistinction to a regression in the service of a new
beginning – one of recognition). I suspect that his diagnosis in this case reflects his
respect for Breuer. There are too many variables in the case to make such a negative judgment.

herself by speaking to her, because the darkness inside her head would not be served well by creating a darkness between patient and analyst, i.e., my silence. This area of therapeutic interchange is most open to misunderstanding and probably defies description. Being unable to reproduce a tape of the sessions, I will presume the reader senses that I would not be conducting the sessions as if they were educational classes. Rather, this therapeutic process would be attempting to aid the growth of what Green (1975) calls *the analytic object*. Such an object relations perspective involves more of a mutuality than is usually recognized in classical analysis. In attempting to describe what he means by an analytic object, Green (1975, p. 12a) writes that:

> . . . in the end the real analytic object is neither on the patient's side nor on the analyst's but in the meeting of these two communications in the potential space which lies between them, limited by the setting which is broken at each separation and reconstituted at each new meeting . . . the analyst does not only unveil a hidden meaning. He constructs a meaning which has never been created before the analytic relationship began.

This meaning, which arises out of this particular object relations situation, i.e., from the interface of this particular patient with this particular analyst, is an essential normative factor in aiding the patient's personal integration and personalization. I would speak, therefore, more than one might expect in a classical analysis, because I would be speaking to the early mothering environment, alluded to above and still present within Anna, which, in its presumptive absence (or intrusive presence), was the context for this child's mind slipping into darkness and for the splitting in her experience of personal integration evidenced by a failure to speak.[4] Whether historically (when Anna was a young child) the mother's presence was one still beclouded by mourning for her lost child, or her mother's presence was that of an intrusive disciplinarian, the effect could be the same, namely these would be cumulative interruptions in her personal sense of continuity of being.

Anywhere from 6 to 8 months into the treatment I could let the couch, the regularity of appointments, the office, and my presence do

---

4 Breuer (in Breuer and Freud, 1893–1895) notes, for example, that Anna 'lost the power of speech (a) as a result of fear, after her first hallucination at night, (b) after having suppressed a remark another time (by active inhibition), (c) after having been unjustly blamed for something and (d) on every analogous occasion (when she felt mortified)' (p. 40).

more of the holding in terms of the good mothering environment, thereby allowing my own comments increasingly to recede into the background. But of silence and of listening, of clarifying and of repeating, it is hard to write, particularly without the living patient. Psychoanalysis is a humanistic science; we interact with people and not with diagnostic categories. I emphasize this in order to put in context the apparent exclusive verbalizations that the literary format of this presentation might lead one to believe would occur.

In addition to the issues of integration and personalization, we can hypothesize obvious disciplinary difficulties, as mentioned above, in Anna's early environment. Of course a child is not a *tabula rasa* upon which the environment simply writes a message for better or ill, because a child's innate biological and psychic mechanisms actively respond to what they are given. In the course of her development, Anna probably did have great difficulty holding together good-mother-loved, bad-mother-feared, anywhere from 18 months on. It is only, as mentioned above, when a child can go from relating to an object to using an object that the successful coming together of a person happens, and we can presume that Anna's later symptomatology betrays that this was not successfully accomplished, i.e., Anna never experienced, as a very young person, that mother world could survive her hatred and come back, after a while, not only surviving but also smiling. In this regard, Winnicott (1971, p. 89) notes:

> In the sequence one can say that first there is object-relating, then in the end there is object-use; in between, however, is the most difficult thing, perhaps, in human development; or most irksome of all the early failures that come for mending. This thing that there is in between relating and use is the subject's placing of the object outside the area of the subject's omnipotent control; that is, the subject's perception of the object as an external phenomenon, not as a projective entity, in fact recognition of it as an entity in its own right.

Summarizing, Winnicott (1971, p. 94) notes one of the positive developmental functions of aggression in the service of personal integration when he says:

> Study of this problem involves a statement of the positive value of destructiveness. The destructiveness, plus the object's survival of the destruction, places the object outside the area of objects set up by the subject's projective mental mechanisms. In this way a world of shared reality is created which the subject can use and which can feed back other-than-me substance into the subject.

Such a resolution of love and hate, we might note, is not only a developmental process but also an experience healing any previous interruptions in the sense of one's continuity of being. The analysis, as we have indicated, would be structured so as to foster such a resolution coming about by means of a regression, which would unravel the primitive thoughts and feelings that were the force behind Anna's splitting of her experience of herself into good and bad, sane and mad, past and present.

Before Anna O.'s resolution of these issues, she would manifest what is referred to as part-object identifications. This is confirmed and exemplified by another one of Anna's symptoms, namely her hallucination that her hair and fingers were black snakes. This hallucination clearly suggests Medea, the murderous mother, and therefore I would use it as an associative backdrop for listening to Anna. (A possible fantasy of Anna's: *Who killed my oldest sister?*) The murderous mother is the unused mother, the not-separated-from mother, and, therefore, the frightening mother-self – the part-object mother, not whole and integrated. This merged with aggressor mother, the person who took care of her and her older dead sisters. All of these aspects of the murderous mother fantasy, not merely its possible occurrence, would be explored.

Having explained to Anna that there were leftover fears from childhood about the death of her sister, that the unintegrated good self and bad self were understandable phenomena having to do with a progressive integration of herself in dialogue with the mother environment, and that a break in one's sense of continuity of being would give rise, in adulthood, to a fear of madness to come and to a subjective sense of a great inner darkness – having said all this, in a context of respect for this troubled person, I would expect noticeable alleviation of symptoms and, more importantly, growth in her experience of personal aliveness. Only when, however, the isolation of her inner darkness could be overcome, and here we are talking about a considerable amount of therapeutic time, could Anna begin to resolve the hysteria of her symptoms, those manic distractions, and resume the developmentally aborted task of finding out and creating whom she was as a person.

Needless to say, this work should markedly improve Anna's condition.[5] If the treatment went well, the patient would gradually allow a

---

5 Sometime during the first year, as a general practice, I would have requested a
  physical examination to rule out any organicity.

more basic, more primitive level of dependency to come to the fore in reference to the analyst. Thus, one could conjecture that the subsequent death of her father, while being experienced as a serious event, would not have to precipitate a destructive psychic withdrawal. Given the regressive context of the treatment, I believe Anna would talk about her pain as well as cry for her lost lover father. The lover aspect would clear up eventually, I believe, but not solely by an interpretation of an oedipal involvement. Seeing whether it cleared up this apparent oedipal issue would test the validity of a pre-oedipal interpretation, i.e., I would say to Anna that she most likely used her relationship with her father for defensive purposes via over-idealization and over-identification, to ward off her part-object bad mother. (This defensive process might explain why she had done so well in school and why she may have been particularly frustrated with her life at home and jealous of her brother.) Although there was probably a sexualization of this defensive process, Anna's pathology had more to do with her relationship with her mother than with an oedipal attachment to her father. The role of father would then be understood not so much as an oedipal figure but rather the needed father person of childhood who protects against the bad witch Medea (the split-off part-object mother). If this line of thought were correct, and Anna was able to hear it, she would be able to allow more primitive fantasies to emerge in analysis. Addressing another of Anna's symptoms, I would say to her that what was important to remember was not only the incident of a dog drinking from her glass but the fact that this may well have signified for her a breaking into a civilized mode of life of primitive unintegrated oral aggression, the oral aggression of the bad-mother-witch.

As mentioned above, if this line of thought and interpretation were correct, Anna would not get markedly worse at the death of her father. Furthermore, having talked to the angry self of childhood who did not know what to do with her aggression, Anna would not have to be hospitalized, because some of her severe splitting would have been alleviated. If a feeling of safety in the analysis were internalized, she would not have to conduct her own analysis, e.g., by stating the date when she would be cured. Rather, she could let the analyst and analysis serve as a needed protective shell enabling the darkness inside her to be confronted and not manically fled from, via her symptoms. Thus, Anna's symptoms would be understood not primarily as mnemic symbols of particular traumatic experiences, as Freud (1910) postulates, but as attempts to cope (in a manic way) with the deadness of the dark space within her. By the analytic process, Anna would be attempting to reach *a new beginning*, to use Balint's (1979) term. This would occur if she were able to remain in treatment and tolerate the encounter, via transferences, with the bad-mother-self without deteriorating repetitively into re-enacting split-off love/hate object relations.[6] As the darkness within her began to resolve itself, the frantic quality of her symptoms, with their strong narcissistic hysterical flavor, could be dealt with more directly by saying to Anna that such frantic maneuvers, *her splitting*, were a distraction from the *madness* within her. Furthermore, her symptoms perpetuated an experience of herself that incapacitated her in handling aggression. In addition, I would mention that it was possible to find a way of negotiating life without finding mortification everywhere.

The fundamental issue in my analysis with Anna O. would be how to facilitate her being a real (emotionally alive, centered) person. The treatment today would be guided by the metaphor of the internal journey whereby Anna could find the safe, quiet place from which she could meet the world, with all its frustrations and limitations, without recourse to primitive defenses. Winnicott (1965, p. 189) warns us of certain dangers in this type of work and of the developmental issues involved for the patient when he says:

> More dangerous, however, is the state of affairs in an analysis in which the analyst is permitted by the patient to reach to the deepest layers of the analysand's personality because of his position as subjective object, or because of the dependence of the patient in the transference psychosis; here there is danger if the analyst interprets instead of waiting for the patient to creatively discover. It is only here, at the place when the analyst has not changed over from a subjective object to one that is objectively perceived, that psychoanalysis is dangerous, and the danger is one that can be avoided if we know how to behave ourselves. If we wait we become objectively perceived in the patient's own time, but if we fail to behave in a way that is facilitating the patient's analytic process . . . we suddenly become not-me for the patient, and then we know too much and we are dangerous because we are too nearly in communication with the central still and silent spot of the patient's ego organization.

---

6 Such deterioration would indicate what Balint calls a malignant regression, whereas a capacity to tolerate what had been said to her in the service of experiencing and overcoming the darkness would indicate a regression in the service of recognition.

The other side of this quiet spot, as I have mentioned above, is madness, the madness that comes from repetitive impingements on one's sense of continuity of being and being taken care of, prerequisites to integration and personalization. In aiming at the darkness in Anna's head, and the self behind the split selves she showed to the world, we would be attempting to get to the deepest elements of her personality. Winnicott (1958, p. 100) notes, for example:

> The analysis of the hysteric (popular term) is the analysis of the madness that is feared but which is not reached without the provision of a new example of infant care, better infant care in the analysis than was provided at the time of the patient's infancy. But please note the analysis does and must get to the madness, although the diagnosis remains neurosis, not psychosis.

To elaborate the case any further without the actual Anna O. is too speculative to be pursued. I have discussed some of the major themes that would preoccupy my thinking in working with an Anna O. Of course, what would actually occur in the spontaneity of the meeting of the patient with the analyst is impossible to predict. The actual treatment flows from such a living relationship. In the tone of voice or body movement, the patient can be telling the analyst that no interpretations, no matter how correct, can be heard, or, on the other hand, a signal can be given that something must be said. Sometimes the minor bodily movements of the analyst, as Musad Khan (1974) has written, will affect the patient's capacity to use a particular session.

I have attempted to show where the analysis might go, following some of the themes of the English object relations school. To say that we might, in following this approach, be seeing farther than Breuer and Freud is not a statement of their limitations but rather of their achievements. That Breuer was perhaps overly frightened by an eroticized transference is not evidence of an intellectual or characterological timidity; that Freud was not so frightened, in his work with similar cases, can be understood as his having had the time and perspective to reflect on Breuer's experience. His vantage point was different, and so he handled things in a different way. The primary danger for analysts today would not be a possible eroticized transference/countertransference reaction but rather the analyst's over-activity via interpretations, hindering the patient from finding the quiet center within the self, with all the madness that might be involved in such a journey. For the analyst to allow the patient to find his or her madness is for the analyst to allow such madness to be re-found in him- or herself. Winnicott has cautioned analysts repeatedly about ignoring that quiet, centered, solitary place out of which one arises as an emotionally alive person, in their haste to do and figure out all kinds of *therapeutic* things. In Anna O.'s case, only when one can get beyond any symptom appraisal of the situation do the dynamics become clear. That Anna accomplished as much as she did with her life is testimony that she got more from Breuer than he indicates.[7] That she had to write, as Ellenberger (1970) indicates, so many of her own obituaries at the end of her life, so obsessively, means there was still a part of her that was lost and that Anna was looking for, right up until her death. The question remains, have we found Anna O.?

---

7 Notwithstanding all the serious limitations of Breuer's treatment, it is obvious that he was a good object for Anna O.; he spent many hours with her, gave her a good deal of personal attention, and genuinely wished her well. He was a concerned authority figure in her life – while her father was dying.

SECTION 3
D.W. WINNICOTT

Chapter 10

Winnicott's psychoanalytic playground

We live in this world when we love it.

Rabindranath Tagore (1949/1977, p. 258)

Man and culture

It might seem odd that D.W. Winnicott (1971), in *Playing and Reality*, quotes the Hindu poet Rabindranath Tagore as a backdrop for his psychoanalytic reflections. But, as one gets to know the man, the choice, it is clear, is not odd at all. Tagore (1949/1977) muses on the countless cycles of life whereas Winnicott invites us down to the seas, to the timeless sand, and reminds us that, if we are to experience the world as interesting, worthwhile, and fertile, play must go from a theoretical possibility to a personal experience.[1,2] What this means for the practice of psychoanalysis, however, is still being explored. Freud's concern that his reflections and observations be classified as science still casts its shadow over our theoretical formulations and everyday practice.[3] Winnicott's appeal is the result of the promise he holds out that an analyst can do credible work without sacrificing individual creativity and spontaneity.

---

1 Tagore writes: 'On the seashores of endless worlds children play' (1949/1977, p. 14).
2 Winnicott states that 'psychotherapy is done in the overlap of the two play areas, that of the patient and that of the therapist. If the therapist cannot play, then he is not suitable for the work. If the patient cannot play, then something needs to be done to enable the patient to become able to play, after which psychotherapy may begin' (1971, p. 54). He also writes that 'psychoanalysis has been developed as a highly specialized form of playing in the service of communication with oneself and others' (1971, p. 41).
3 See Winnicott D.W. (1989). Note Winnicott's review of Jung's memoirs: 'if I want to say that Jung was mad, and that he recovered, I am doing nothing worse than I would do in saying of myself that I was sane and that through analysis and self-analysis I achieved some measure of insanity. Freud's flights to sanity could be something we psychoanalysts are trying to recover from' (p. 483).

Although clearly acknowledging the import of subjective phantasy, Winnicott stands in the philosophical tradition that presumes that human beings make contact and interact with the objective communal world, i.e., what we are capable of knowing is reality itself, that which stands in the shadow of internal phantasy, but which is knowable as objective. Consequently object relations, as applicable to Winnicott, is not a special brand of intrapsychic discourse (not a descriptive term for internal imagoes) but rather an obvious statement about our essential communal make-up. Our selves are formed by everything that comes to pass between us, everything that constitutes our personal and/or social history. Human beings do not have relationships; they are relationships. No meaningful analytic work can be done without that awareness.

In contradistinction to other analytic thinkers, Winnicott was not concerned with structuring a formalized psychoanalytic theory of humans. To read Winnicott is not to enter the arena of logical argumentation, but rather to experience an invitation to muse and to create along with him. Ever desirous of encouraging personal spontaneity and creativity, he was reluctant to codify his approach lest the very qualities he deemed essential for human life be rigidified through submission to a *knowing other*.[4] Instead he spoke, almost casually, about the route we humans must travel in our task of achieving personal maturation, the necessary processes we need to traverse in order to step outside the circle of mother– self–world to find the wider circle of the world of self and other. Such a world is one in which we are destined to spend our lives with a sense of either personal aliveness or conforming deadness.

Play, as we know, belongs to personal aliveness and therefore presumes that an individual has come together into a usable self. The process of *coming together as a person* was, for Winnicott, intrinsic to his understanding of people. He studied the ingredients, as it were, that enabled humans to be capable of love and hate, of recognizing their selves and other selves, those whom we can meet on shared ground – the endless sand – and build a place to be. Winnicott (1971) would eventually call such building creative, and the fruits of such labor the gifts of culture. But to step into the circle of culture is, in Winnicott's thought, to re-find the *transitional space* of early childhood, that overlapping area, that gentle mixture of self and other – the

---

4   Roustang (1982) writes, 'If the analyst relies entirely on himself in practice, he cannot rely on someone else in theory. To dissociate the two makes no sense, because theorization can take place only during practice' (p. 72).

world, as it were, waiting to be found with all of a person's history active in the searching. All such finding is, of necessity, a creating.

To be alive means that the overlapping circle of personal illusion and objective reality (the seedbed of culture) is experienced as likable and entertaining, inviting as well as challenging.[5] As teddy bears negotiate a child's many selves, for example, the world is put to new and personal uses, and culture is fertilized.

Winnicott (1971) considered psychoanalysis as one of the primary inheritors of the transitional space of childhood play, i.e., one of the cultural outcomes of a good-enough childhood; he thought of it alongside such other achievements as art, philosophy, and religion – bridges, all of them. They are, in Winnicott's thought, links between our insides (forgotten as well as remembered), and the world around us, between the *me* and the *not me*.[6] In the creation of culture, we weave the *not me* with our subjective phantasies and produce a world in which we feel safe enough to play. In experiencing ourselves as giving and receiving, the very world that defines us as human comes to be. And so Winnicott (1971) writes that 'cultural experiences are in direct continuity with play, the play of those who have not yet heard of games' (p. 100).

Another avenue Winnicott (1958) offers us, I believe, for exploring his notion of transitional space is to reflect on his concept of mind. Winnicott denies the existence of mind as some type of Leibnitzian monad, as an entity inside one's head.[7] (He was clearly reacting to one psychoanalytic model, influenced by both Descartes and Kant, which locates mind and meaning as locked within the individual psyche.[8]) One fruitful way to read Winnicott's thoughts on psyche/soma is to speak of mind as a personal referent term for a communal accomplishment, i.e., communication in all its possibilities. Language, for

---

5 'We experience life in the area of transitional phenomena, in the exciting interweave of subjectivity and objective observations, and in an area that is intermediate between the inner reality of the individual and the shared reality of the world that is external to individuals' (Winnicott, 1971, p. 64).

6 'The intermediate area to which I am referring is the area that is allowed to the infant between primary creativity and objective perception based on reality testing . . . The mother's adaptation to the infant's needs, when good enough, gives the infant the illusion that there is an external reality that corresponds to the infant's own capacity to create' (Winnicott, 1958, p. 239).

7 'In the study of a developing individual the mind will often be found to be developing a false entity and a false localization' (Winnicott, 1958, p. 244).

8 'Freud draws here a radical distinction between the internal and subjective world, which we can know, and the real, external world, which he claims we cannot . . . So Freud is led to the traditionalist's skeptical view that all knowledge begins and ends with first-person experience' (Cavell, 1993, p. 19).

example, is one such experience of communication enabling us to experience and create mind.[9] Such communication is the building block of our human legacy, to be in a place with others. Such is the task of being alive, and, clearly, such is the goal of analysis. *Human meaning* comes about, consequently, as a result of a shared environment, within a particular cultural context. Although *mind as community* was not a specific turn of phrase for Winnicott, it does reflect what I believe is an essential implication of his approach, i.e., appreciating humans as creative and, consequently, creating a shared culture. Lewis Thomas (1984), the scientist and essayist, has written persuasively of people as constituted by their human communities and not as separate entities definable in terms of self-regulating mechanisms.[10] To isolate the psyche in terms of drives and phantasies, forces and counterforces is to reduce spontaneity to reflex, creativity to formula, and culture to control.

To be alive, for Winnicott, means more than being a compliant response to a particular environment – the triumph, all too frequently, of a false self-organization. Alive is more than mere sanity and clearly some steps beyond instinctual satisfaction.[11] Instincts are understood, in Winnicott's thoughts, as fortifiers for an existent ego, i.e., for the individual who has achieved personal integration.[12] Otherwise drives are experienced as *persecutory-like intrusions*, and their satisfaction a guarantee of nothing more than physical stimulation.[13] Only when we feel personally alive can relationships be humanly satisfying. Grounded in our capacity both to hear and to respond to others, instinctual gratifications have a chance to be personally fulfilling, enabling us to experience that we are not lost stars in an endless night but, in fact, tied to each other by the need to feel real, desired, imaginative, and responsive. Winnicott's therapeutic

---

9 'For an interpersonal or third person view, on the contrary, meanings are not in the head . . . but adhere to thoughts, ideas, and proposition, in virtue of their relationship to this community, to the history of their use, to events and things in the world, and to other ideas' (Cavell, 1988, p. 597).

10 '. . . we get along together in human society because we are genetically designed to be social animals, and we are obliged, by instructions from our genes, to be useful to each other' (Thomas, 1984, p. 104).

11 'Through artistic expression we can hope to keep in touch with our primitive selves whence the most intense feelings and even fearfully acute sensations derive, and we are poor indeed if we are only sane' (Winnicott, 1958, p. 150n).

12 'It is the self that must precede the self's use of instinct' (Winnicott, 1971, p. 141).

13 '. . . but id-excitements can be traumatic when the Ego is not yet able to include them' (Winnicott, 1965, p. 141).

hope is that, as we aid in the process of personal integration, we are not merely contributing to an individual acceptance of *Ananke,* but to a careful building of the human enterprise.

Only when we feel effective in our personal interactions, rather than perpetually accommodating, can aggression be experienced as a stabilizing force for our personal identity and sexuality, a pleasurable securing of the *me* and the *not me.* In the moments of self-forgetful orgasm of self and other, just as in the great cultural achievements of humans, we are allowed to give up the experience of separateness – one might say the *delusion* of separateness. Adult autonomy has more to do with a capacity to depend on and interact with others than it does to function independently. Not only does creativity enter psychoanalytic diagnostic categories but also a capacity for civility, because civility has to do with the careful treatment of others, a maturational achievement that reflects something of what Winnicott means by *using* the object, which is recognizing the other's separateness and interacting accordingly.[14] To be civilized means to live cooperatively in a world of others. An analysis that results in anything less has not reached its goal.

The therapeutic place

Winnicott believed that most parents, particularly mothers, not only had their child's best interest at heart but were also equipped to foster their child's maturational processes.[15] When all did not go well, however, the resolution of such developmental tasks, for either child or adult, became the focus of therapy. As analyst, Winnicott grew convinced that only an individual who could give and receive the rewards of play had fulfilled the potential of creativity that is the mark of a true self-organization. Progressively, throughout his writings, he saw the goal of treatment as enabling a patient to be in a place where such play was possible, where the ebb and flow of life would be both accepted and lived. Not insignificantly does he quote Tagore, a poet who spoke of the utter and complete unity of all things, especially the

---

14 *Accordingly* is, of course, the point. 'To do this is to be freed from the search for the all-powerful knowing Other. When one is no longer subject to the transference desire, one is able to live freely and creatively in the world. Freud was not Reichian when he said the goal of analysis was to be able to love and to work; nor do I think he was, in using the word love, arguing for a delusional state' (Gargiulo, 1989, p. 159).

15 '. . . what we need are mothers (and fathers) . . . who have found out how to believe in themselves. These (parents) build the best homes' (Winnicott, 1957, p. 42).

interdependence of life and death. In the drama of human life, play and illusion (*Lila* and *Maya*) formed the backdrop to both Tagore's and Winnicott's reflections.

Winnicott (1958) made of his psychoanalytic office a transitional space – something contributed to by both analyst and patient, a common playground where they might both meet and create a world, as it were, precisely because there would be a world there to be found. Sometimes that world would have small beginnings: drawing squiggles, by turns, on a piece of paper, for example. Squiggle games were one way Winnicott (1971) found of coming together with a patient and finding a new way of speaking, a unique creation. And finding a new tongue by which to speak of the paradoxes of human existence is to make of the psychoanalytic encounter a place where creativity enters technique, the experience of which is as important for an analyst as it is for a patient. One does not, consequently, just *undergo* an analysis, nor does one simply *conduct* an analysis. One has to be developing all the time a place where memory can be trusted, aloneness can be safe, and love and hate can be traveled repeatedly without any loss of direction. Analysis, then, depends on who is doing it, just as each work of prose, or of poetry, depends on who is doing it – and this does no violence to literary rules or tradition.

Although there is a body of knowledge about human experience and maturation that is essential to a practitioner, each analyst is, as we know, as distinctive a guide as a Virgil to a Dante. Who, therefore, is doing an analysis determines whether it is a stale repetition of formulae or a personalized embodiment of psychoanalytic principles. Winnicott, as the analyst and as the poet that he was, had no interest in establishing a school of thought, no interest, as I have mentioned, in codifying his reflections into a teaching. He was opposed, for example, to Melanie Klein's insistence that her followers use her terms. Such insistence, he felt, would rob the individual practitioner of the chance to find his or her own words for what was going on.[16]

Clinical perspectives

An individual's achieving personal aliveness was, for Winnicott, the linchpin for his or her reflections on human pathology as well as his

---

16 Robert Rodman (1990, p. 33) argued, in 'Insistence on being himself', that 'this artificially integrated phenomenon must be attacked destructively'.

or her therapeutic focus. The resolution of intrapsychic conflict was subordinate to this goal. We live through all kinds of experiences growing up, most of which we cannot hold in our hands but which, nevertheless, we carry with us all our lives. Winnicott knew, particularly because of his work with children, that, when the therapeutic playground was safe, an analyst could help a patient bring to light what had been condemned to darkness, or bring into full view what had been looked at from aside. As patient and analyst experienced continuity they could begin to experience contiguity; standing on level ground they could gradually allow for the play of metaphor, the work of knowing and not knowing, the paradox of love and hate, life and death – the repetitive road marks of an analytic encounter. And in the amiability that could follow from such activity, what had been eclipsed could emerge, what was sidetracked in personal development could begin healing, and even what was missing in the analyst's understanding and approach could be supplied.

It becomes obvious, I believe, why Winnicott would not, could not, organize a school. He merely reminds us what each person, in the analytic meeting, brings to the place of therapy. And on this *ground* there is no automatic indication that an analysis has begun, certainly not the use of the couch. As a patient's contribution to the analytic space is crucial, Winnicott highlighted the need for an analyst not to intrude, or to interpret too early, or, for that matter, too correctly. One safeguard against this last possibility is, I believe, for an analyst to allow him- or herself the experience of forgetting. There are rules to the play, but one must frequently forget prior experiences and expectations if the present is not to be overshadowed by too much thinking or too much need for an analyst to be in the know as to what is happening.[17]

The patient

For all of Winnicott's understanding of the observable developmental stages, he never lost sight of the complexity of the human situation. As

---

17 Winnicott (1965, p. 189) writes, 'I have always felt that an important function of interpretation is the establishment of the limits of the analyst's understanding'. He also wrote: 'It does not really matter, of course, how much the therapist knows provided he can hide his knowledge' (Winnicott, 1971, p. 57). Winnicott is indicating the need for an analyst never to violate a patient's inner core – that center from which the true self-organization springs.

easily as he can speak of the good-enough mother's adaptation to her child's needs, he can speak of the necessary, although hidden, role of illusion in a child's coming to be – illusion, that is, as the subjective phantasy whereby a child creates the world, the satisfier of his or her needs, as a first and necessary step in dialoguing with the other.[18] When the other, usually the mother, meets such phantasies with her own responsiveness, the world is experienced as giving and welcoming, and so a child can engage it with minimal anxiety. And that engagement means that a person finds that he or she is not alone, no solitary island, lost. Winnicott's thoughts are clear: dialogue with the world, personally and culturally, is what should define human experience. Erik Erikson speaks in the same vein when he notes that, from a more observational stance, both mother and child truly do create each other in their different roles. When the mother is able to experience the child as her own, responsive to his or her individual timings, as well as be created by the child as his or her own, we have the first dance of reciprocity, from which civility and culture follow. When this does not occur, personal integration gets sidetracked and rage and desolation roam the psyches of both caretaker and cared for, and the experience of personal aliveness is either aborted or eclipsed.

In such circumstances, Winnicott would interview both mother and child; he would employ the whole family, if necessary, to find the thread of personal ongoing in being which had been sidetracked into reactive compliance or defiant isolation. He would proceed so because, when things had gone badly, a child's personal history was all too often a chronology of objective environmental misalignments. And what had occurred in childhood was Winnicott's lens through which he understood adult patients as well. Such developmental misalignments would issue, all too easily, in hatred coming to the fore, not the hatred that psychically kills the other, just as it delights in its resurrection (which we will speak of later when discussing his thoughts on reparation and concern), but an angry disjunction between the self and the world. He would come to speak of this as the *antisocial*

---

18 'It will be seen that fantasy is not something the individual creates to deal with external reality's frustrations. This is only true of fantasying. Fantasy is more primary than reality, and the enrichment of fantasy with the world's riches depends on the experience of illusion' (Winnicott, 1958, p. 153). Note also Winnicott's statement that 'fantasying interferes with action and with life in the real or external world, but much more so it interferes with dream and with the personal or inner psychic reality, the living core of the individual personality' (Winnicott, 1971, p. 31). Therefore, my spelling of the word phantasy.

tendency.[19] Hatred eventually acknowledged, however, is one of the important steps toward personal integration; hatred understood is not just lethal it is already receding to make way for some usable personal contact. The raged-at world can become the usable world, just as the raged-at analyst can become usable also. Angry disjunctures are not easy to work with and so Winnicott (1958) could talk of his own response of hatred to a patient that he might hold in isolation until a patient could hear of it and the hearing could be helpful.[20]

When things have gone badly in Eden, when the world has been found short of being good enough, other symptoms, as we have spoken about, come to the fore. The transitional space between the child and his or her personal world becomes garbled and the precursor of mind, as communication, is aborted. The child, or adult, is forced to retreat into his or her own ruminations, back into observation rather than response, back into fearful, skewed perceptions reacting to an environment more with compliance than with spontaneity – a compliance that is the forerunner of what Winnicott calls the false self, as against spontaneity, the hallmark of a true self-organization.

When the stage is cluttered with deadening experiences – impulses that have lost a personal grounding, memories that eclipse the self – a person has no alternative but to re-enact such a history, repeatedly, with all those with whom he or she comes in contact. Transference, then, is an inability to find new lines for the play of our lives. The old lines are repeated and defended as a person tries to author him- or herself with a script that is not his or her own. It is as if the dead of the past outnumber the living present, as if one is having a dialogue with masks.[21] In the new speech, the new language between analyst and patient, and the new hearing, the voices of the past can find a resting place.

Winnicott was content to limit himself to a few comments during a session; he understood and was comfortable communicating that he

19 'The antisocial tendency is characterized by an element in it which compels the environment to be important. The patient through unconscious drives compels someone to attend to management. It is the task of the therapist to become involved in this the patient's unconscious drive'. Also: 'The antisocial tendency implies hope' (Winnicott, 1958, p. 309).

20 Winnicott writes, 'In analysis of psychotics the analyst is under greater strain to keep his hate latent, and he can only do this by being thoroughly aware of it . . . If the patient (however) seeks objective or justified hate he must be able to reach it, else he cannot feel he can reach objective love' (1958, p. 199).

21 By way of analogy, note Calvino's observation (1974, p. 75): 'You reach a moment in life when . . . the dead outnumber the living. And the mind refuses to accept more faces . . . on every new face . . . it prints the old forms, for each one it finds the most suitable mask'.

was, at times, the patient's father or mother. No need for psychotic labels, just history unfolding. The play of transference, however, is more than allowing and clarifying its occurrence; its resolution is fostered only within a context of an analyst's personal presence, one that is neither confessional nor intimate, but available, sensible, and concerned – a presence, I believe, that knows how important it is to convey to patients that we are as committed to holding their dreams as we are to interpreting them.

The therapist

Winnicott (1965, p. 163) speaks of countertransference as the lack of professionalism in how one conducts oneself vis-à-vis a patient. One example of professionalism, in Winnicott's context of the psychoanalytic encounter, is the therapist's appreciation of the developmental needs of a patient and the fostering of their integration. Developmental needs, in the task of personal integration (personalization and realization), are, by definition, different from instinctual gratifications. As he knew the significance of this distinction, Winnicott (1971) was not anxious when providing milk and cookies, for example, for those patients for whom he thought it would be helpful. He wrote, also, of rocking a particularly regressed patient in his arms until there was a quiet, personal experience of breathing, enabling the patient thereby to touch the ground of his or her life, so to speak.[22] He had extended sessions for those people who were not able to get to his office with the usual frequency. And he was quite content to let a patient come upon an inexact interpretation, which might be close enough to the mark, rather than offer, even presuming he knew it, the correct interpretation himself.

Thus, it becomes clearer that *who* is doing the work is no call to wild analysis but rather awareness that the psychoanalytic encounter is as distinctive as good prose, or as personally affirming and consoling as the best of poetry. And just as a land without a bard is desolate, so the psychoanalytic place is empty if it is filled, as I have mentioned, with correct formulae rather than personal experiences. In this sense

---

22 'Treatment is needed, rather than technique, and intuitive behavior and management, not verbal interpretations' (Little, 1990, p. 88). 'Through his reliable holding (Winnicott, 1952b) and acceptance of a direct relationship, I began to trust D.W. and to find continuity and something of a mutual feeding situation (Winnicott, 1970b)' (Little, 1990, p. 98).

Winnicott stands in the tradition of the experimental work of Sandor Ferenczi (1988), although likewise fulfilling the analytic task so ably described by Andre Green (1975). Green reminds us that simply to repeat what has been handed down to us would be effectively to kill analysis; keeping this knowledge alive and vital means innovation.[23] And innovation is only possible when one can trust one's good will toward a patient as well as trusting one's good will toward oneself, in order to indulge in enough forgetfulness to be surprised, in Theodor Reik's (1948) sense, by what may transpire[24] – a forgetfulness that is close to what Freud (1913) meant by free hovering attention. Self-awareness can be, all too easily, a by-product of the anxious ego, a hindrance to inventiveness.

And Winnicott was inventive. Some of his interventions are open to conflicting interpretations. Yet for him, I am certain, rocking a patient in the hope that some primal memory would be touched, and the disruption in the patient's personal experience of ongoing-in-being resumed, was not seen as either seductive or harmful. With goodwill toward oneself, an analyst need not be totally right in his or her interpretations in order to avoid being totally wrong. And one might even have as a goal, in conveying an interpretation to particular patients, that they would experience the limitations of their analyst's understanding. Winnicott did.

Countertransference, for Winnicott, as we have mentioned, is anything that interferes with an analyst's professional stance. In this vein, Masud Khan (1975, p. xxviii) suggests that analysts frequently see their patients as more integrated than they, in fact, are – in order that they might experience themselves functioning as analysts, i.e., for example, conducting an analysis, for years, on the 'false assumption that the patient is alive' (Winnicott, 1965, p. 152). This means, I believe, that when pathology has had the upper hand we have the experience of mind as a solipsistic entity, a locked-in-ness, so to speak, which comes about when an individual has had to take over the protective functions that should have been provided by his or her caring environment. The

---

23 Green states that 'an analyst cannot practice psychoanalysis and keep it alive by applying knowledge. He must attempt to be creative to the limits of his ability' (1975, p. 18a). He also argues that 'In the end the real analytic object is neither on the patient's side nor on the analyst's but in the meeting of these two communications in the potential space which lies between them . . . , the analyst . . . constructs a meaning which has never been created before the analytic relationship began' (Green, 1975, p. 12a).

24 'On the threshold of psychological research we find, not familiarity with ourselves, but astonishment at the phenomena of our own minds' (Reik, 1948, p. 239).

individual becomes, consequently, both caretaker and cared for, overly self-conscious and apprehensively cautious – the caretaker-self, caught, in a hall of mirrors. When such a turn of events comes to be, obsessive ruminations predominate and the capacity for playful metaphorical interchange is eclipsed. When a patient is locked into his or her mind, and not at home in his or her soma, we have the breeding ground of an analysis lasting for years but getting nowhere. In such cases, Winnicott would search beyond the rubble of intellectual awareness for what was life giving, be it a patient's need to find forgotten rage and/or protective (managerial) care in order to begin a personal self.[25,26]

Winnicott, as we have mentioned, reminds analysts that a patient must learn to play first before any productive investigative or clarifying process can be undertaken. Squiggling games can be done with more than lines on a paper; they can be done with words that need not issue in anything more than moments of basic trust. A human life is made of such moments. It is against such a backdrop that we can understand Winnicott's hope that death would find him *alive*.[27]

A case in point

Let us conjure up a case he wrote about. A man, somewhere in his mid-40s, comes to his office, a man who has tried analysis for the past 25 years with different analysts. He is a successful man, by many worldly standards, but a man unable to resolve a persistent feeling that all is not well within. With such a case, Winnicott allowed himself to suspend his own perceptions, because he trusted himself, and to say to the patient that, although he knew the patient was male, he heard a female in the room, he saw a female in the room. And to complete the circle he told the patient, what would eventually prove integral to his previous comments, that he, Winnicott, of course, knew that he was mad for saying this. Not metaphor; Winnicott's *madness*, he would later assure the patient, was but a moment of suspended perception, in order to contact a hidden experience that the patient was unknowingly carrying

25 'If, in the fantasy of early growth, there is contained death, then at adolescence there is contained murder . . . In the unconscious fantasy, growing up is inherently an aggressive act' (Winnicott, 1971, p. 144).

26 'In the third grouping I place all those patients whose analyses must deal with the early stages of emotional development [when] . . . the personal structure is not yet securely founded . . . the accent is more surely on management' (Winnicott, 1958, p. 279).

27 See C. Winnicott (1989, p. 4): 'Oh God! May I be alive when I die.'

around. What conjectured experience? That his mother, now dead, during the earliest periods of his life, saw a girl, out of her own madness, before she was able to handle and see her son as male.

One foot in the past, eyes toward the future, hopes grounded in timeless, mostly hidden images, our namable selves reflect how we were called, how we were spoken to. Winnicott's patient had been spoken to as if he were a girl every time his mother interacted with him during his earliest months, and the confusion as to who he was, who he was supposed to be, echoed through his life. Content to think that in many cases poetic listening was more helpful than diagnostic categories, Winnicott could let his mind wander to a place where we all may be confused as to who we are, or are supposed to be. And reaching such a place in himself, without repudiation, he could hear the echo of that little girl in the consultation room and name it for his patient (Winnicott, 1971, pp. 72–75).

Self, other, and the world

Individuals are not so much alone as lonely until another hears them, with his or her whole self, as it were. Only then can the potential transitional space between oneself and what is not oneself become actual. And by actual Winnicott means something analogous to a bridge being built, a co-creation between a child and the mothering environment, between analyst and patient – a co-creation where what is created is also simply found, creation meaning finding it for oneself. And finding the world for oneself, making it a real place where spontaneity is possible, is an essential prologue to what we call the work of human hands, the world of culture – in traditional psychoanalytic language, the world of sublimation; not the sublimation of certain people at special moments, however, but the everyday creation of the alive-enough person.[28]

How important, then, is Winnicott's therapeutic focus on enabling a patient to feel personally alive, because without such experience the world is a dead place. It is with such a goal of aliveness in mind that

28 'We can understand sublimation, consequently, as closely related, if not identical, to the symbolic use of objects in this place of play, manifested by the capacity to play . . . Ideally, therefore, sublimation starts in the first year and progressively continues throughout an individual's life. It is the capacity to adaptively use symbols at different development levels; that is, in a way that makes play, as Winnicott understands it, possible' (Gargiulo, 1992, p. 32). See Chapter 11 for a more detailed discussion.

Winnicott (1965) explored the roots of childhood phantasy finding there, as a necessary stage, a destruction of the world, which is, para-doxically, a backdrop for experiencing the world as separate, outside of our omnipotent control. Experiencing the world as separate enables a child (or adult) to *use* it, as such, and not simply *relate to* the other as provider.

Experiencing the world as separate means achieving a capacity for reparation – a Kleinian concept that Winnicott made his own. Such a capacity is able to come about, Winnicott wrote, when guilt over a psy-chic killing is held but not felt as such, so that the experience of concern predominates.[29] Reparation and concern are, then, the building blocks of communal civility. Achieving such a developmental capacity establish-es, on firm ground, the child as separate, as aggressive, and as essentially related. As a child goes from relating to the mother-world to developing a capacity to use, i.e., to appreciate as separate, the mother-world, he experiences a gradual change over from unintegration to integration – all of which fosters the experience of being a unique person.[30] Such uniqueness entails, Winnicott (1958, p. 36) notes, not only a 'capacity to be alone' but also an aloneness that comes about through our objective relatedness – alone, that is, in the presence of someone else, alone, also, even to oneself – an aloneness that must be recognized, and not violat-ed, by an analyst.[31] Consequently Winnicott's (1958, p. 137) remark that 'there is no such thing as a baby' (without a mother) is more than a clever phrase, and that there is no such thing as a patient (without an analyst) is more than an obvious implication.[32] They are fundamental statements about human beings, i.e., they are relational by nature, most obviously experienced in the creation and use of language in the service of understanding others, oneself, and the world in which one lives.

Erikson (1966) also spoke of the early dialogue of mother and child as the *ontology of ritualization,* a place where the capacity for the sym-bolic is born (the divided coin, as it were, half mother, half child, the unification of which is both a creation and a re-finding of mother and

---

29 'Failure of reparation leads to a losing of the capacity for concern, and to its replacement by primitive forms of guilt and anxiety' (Winnicott, 1965, p. 82).

30 'So for Winnicott the healthy integration made possible by a holding environment is always reversible; states of unintegration can be tolerated and enjoyed. But if integration is incom-plete or partial the unintegrated parts of the infant become, in Winnicott's view, dissociated' (Phillips, 1988, p. 81).

31 Winnicott (1965, p. 187) writes that 'each individual is an isolate, permanently non-commu-nicating, permanently unknown, in fact unfound'.

32 For a clinical discussion of this approach, see Gargiulo (1991, pp. 155–166).

child, of self and of other).[33,34] The baby creates the mother as mother, i.e., the baby's response, when things go well, evokes motherliness, just as the mother's response, in experiencing the child as her own, creates him or her to her own image. When an individual is not locked in deadly combat for the fulfillment of basic needs, a healthy relationship can predominate. And the capacity for symbolization can begin because mother, as herself, *and* as the found world, is not experienced with terror but rather with possibility.

What possibility? The possibility to come upon, through symbolization, forgotten aspects of the self and/or of the other, of love or hate, of sexuality and/or loss hidden in the world, tucked inside the most common of things or images, transforming the place where we live into a playground for the Muses. Symbolization, and by implication sublimation, are not isolated achievements; they are the consequence of being personally alive and contributing to the communal, dialogic world in which we live[35] – the triumph of play, if you will.

Play, however, is always free, not imposed. Winnicott was convinced that the more we are able to raise children respecting their *person-ness*, the more morality, a necessary prerequisite for living in an adult communal world, would follow. In his thought, quite rightly I believe, the fact that morality is taught, frequently by some external religious authority, is a statement of our still, as yet, inadequate child-rearing practices. In his respect for a person's individuality and internality, Winnicott was essentially a profoundly spiritual man; he was not interested, however, in polemics about religion. Anyone familiar with Zen thought, or Vedantic Hinduism, will hear echoes while reading him, particularly, for example, in his understanding of the role of breathing in establishing a personal soma. (To live in the body is the start of life.) In this vein we can understand Winnicott's reflections on the madness of attempting to impose one's personal world upon another as their necessary world. Such missionizing, he believed, is a violation of sanity and civility. He was not an advocate for missionaries – not religious or political, and particularly not

---

33 Erikson (1966, p. 613) writes: 'In all epigenetic development, however, a ritual element, once evolved, must be progressively reintegrated on each higher level, so that it will become an essential part of all subsequent stages'.

34 'In between the infant and the object is something, or some activity or sensation. In so far as this joins the infant to the object (viz. maternal part-object) so far is this the basis of symbol-formation. On the other hand, in so far as this something separates instead of joins, so is its function of leading on to symbol-formation blocked' (Winnicott, 1965, p. 146).

35 'Winnicott's experience of man as playful (*homo ludens*) enabled him to create a playground where culture and personal consciousness mirror each other' (Gargiulo, 1992, p. 332).

psychoanalytic. There is, we can conclude, madness in possessing the truth. 'A capacity for compromise is not a characteristic of the insane' Winnicott notes (1988, p. 138).[36] Compromise entails not eclipsing, by denial, our solitariness in all its roles, nor our own death in all its epiphanies, avoiding thereby, what Winnicott calls, the manic defence.[37] Compromise is essential if we are to live in ourselves and with others.

Closing thoughts

Winnicott understood, as I read him, that holding one's patients' dreams is a necessary task, so that they can eventually hold them themselves, confident that the world will not let them go until, of course, it is time for them to say good-bye – alive. He preferred to traverse the human landscape rather than simply observe it. Concerned with what it means to be alive, to be in health, he replaced empirical detachment with personal experience. It is a lingering prejudice, in some professional quarters, not to hear this as scientific, as a commitment to understanding, without preconceived notions.[38]

It is not without reason that the ancient Greeks spoke of happiness as residing in the full exercise of personal competence, the same civilization that read nature and told us that love begets love forever. Winnicott, from all appearances, achieved both competence and love, and shared these with us.[39]

We are indebted to his generosity.

---

36 Note the preceding sentence as well: 'If development proceeds well the individual becomes able to deceive, to lie, to compromise, to accept conflict as a fact and to abandon the extreme ideas of perfection and an opposite to perfection that make existence intolerable' (Winnicott, 1988, pp. 137–138). Winnicott also writes, 'When Jung deliberately lied to Freud he became a unit with a capacity to hide secrets instead of a split personality with no place for hiding anything' (Winnicott, 1989, p. 487).

37 Note Winnicott's (1958, pp. 143–144) thoughts on the manic defence, which is 'intended to cover a person's capacity to deny the depressive anxiety that is inherent in emotional development, anxiety that belongs to the capacity of the individual to feel guilt, and also to acknowledge responsibility for instinctual experiences, and for the aggression in the fantasy that goes with instinctual experiences'. Winnicott (1958, pp. 131–132) states, '[It] is characteristic of the manic defence that the individual is unable fully to believe in the liveliness that denies deadness, since he does not believe in his own capacity for object love; for making good is only when the destruction is acknowledged'.

38 Winnicott (1988, p. 574): 'Freud gave us this method which we can use, and it doesn't matter what it leads us to. The point is, it does lead us to things; it's an objective way of looking at things . . . for people who can go to something without preconceived notions, which, in a sense, is science.'

39 Lear (1990, p. 187) notes, 'The creation of the individual and the caring for the individual are of a piece. For it is only with the internalization of these caring relationships that here emerges a creature sufficiently reflective and self-aware to deserve the title of individual'.

CHAPTER 11

Sublimation: Winnicottian reflections[1]

Children have their play on the seashore of worlds.

Rabindranath Tagore (1949/1977, p. 41)

In this chapter, I discuss some of Winnicott's theoretical contributions as they relate to the concept of sublimation. The concept of sublimation, which has been recurrently studied in the classic literature, can be productively enhanced, I believe, by placing it within a Winnicottian object relations framework. I will delineate the classic understanding of sublimation and, of necessity, the corollary concept of symbol formation, in order to provide a background for appreciating Winnicott's particular contributions. I hope to show that Winnicott's ideas and models are pre-eminently useful in trying to grasp what has been an elusive concept in psychoanalytic reflections.

In discussing sublimation, one is addressing cultural achievements, that area of human interaction where we experience ourselves as communicative through such experiences as art, music, religion, philosophy, and, of course, psychoanalysis. Freud, as we know, concentrated primarily on delimiting the intrapsychic terrain, and his formulations consequently reflect this perspective. Winnicott does not repudiate Freud's work but rather looks to a different place in order to understand our cultural heritage. His concept of the transitional area between the *me* and the *not me* became, for him, the playground in which he did a good deal of his musings. This short study focuses on Winnicott's concept of the transitional play space in order to offer a wider context, than the classic Freudian position, for understanding

---

1 This is a revised version of an article that appeared in The Psychoanalytic Review (Gargiulo, 1992).

sublimation, and thereby to gain a deeper appreciation for the cultures we create.[2]

Freud's therapy of uncovering the hidden and bringing to light the *repudiated* reflects his preference for studying what he calls the cellar of the soul, i.e., the individual's unconscious desires and conflicts. His reading of symbol and of sublimation, therefore, conceptualizes them as tributaries of our instinctuality and/or conflicted, related defense mechanisms. In *Civilization and Its Discontents* (Freud, 1930), he speaks of cultural/civilized life as based primarily on the renunciation of instinctual satisfactions. Freud's model of the mind, his metaphorical image of humans, is that of an individual psyche with its various mechanisms for handling sexual and aggressive conflicts. Winnicott, in *Playing and Reality* (1971), speaks about the interaction between mother and child as crucial for understanding the seedbed, so to speak, from which a person grows. He postulates a transitional arena, a potential space where this interaction occurs, a space where both mothering-world and emerging-self set down the rules of their play together. Having brought us to this place, Winnicott has, in effect, given us a different language and therefore a different perspective to understand cultural experiences. Play, Winnicott (1971) reminds us, is always a communal activity, not an individual solipsistic one. 'Only in playing', he writes, 'is communication possible' (p. 54).

Before developing this further, I would like briefly to summarize the traditional understanding of sublimation. To understand Jones' (1948) approach to sublimation, one has to know his theory of symbolism, which he speaks of as follows:

> The symbol is a substitutive, perceptual replacement-expression for something hidden, with which it has evident characteristics in common . . . Its essence lies in its having two or more meanings . . . Its tendency from the conceptual to the perceptual indicates its nearness to primitive thought . . . (p. 96)

> Only what is repressed is symbolized; only what is repressed needs to be symbolized . . . [Symbols are ideas that] are invested in consciousness with a logically inexplicable and unfounded affect, and of which it may be analytically established that they owe this affective over-emphasis to unconscious identification with another idea, to which the surplus of affect really belongs . . . (p. 116)

---

2   For an interesting attempt to update the concept of sublimation with some awareness of relating this concept to the experience of object constancy, see Sandler and Joffee (1987, p. 191 et seq.).

Jones discusses what is repressed and mentions that the range of what is symbolized is relatively limited to early body experiences, such as birth, love, death, sexual functions, and emotional experiences with early parental figures. Various authors have essentially maintained this understanding of symbolization.[3] Ricoeur (1970, p. 505), in *Freud and Philosophy*, states:

> Symbolism in the Freudian sense expressed the failure of sublimation and not its advancement, as Jones readily admits: The affect investing the symbolized ideas has not, insofar as the symbolism is concerned, proved capable of that modification in quality denoted by the term sublimation.

By the words 'that modification in quality', psychoanalysis conceptualized instinctual energy as having a new and different aim.[4] Consequently sublimation, in this context, has been thought of primarily as occasional achievements occurring when an individual reaches beyond basic instinctual satisfactions to experiences that contribute to society.[5]

When one's understanding of sublimation follows the displacement of aim model, a psychoanalytic account of culture is necessarily limited. Laplanche and Pontalis (1973, p. 433) note, for example:

> Because Freud left the theory of sublimation in such a primitive state we have only the vaguest hints as to the dividing-lines between sublimation and processes akin to it (reaction formation, aim-inhibition, idealization, repression). Similarly, although Freud held the capacity to sublimate to be an essential factor in successful treatment, he never described its operation in concrete terms . . . The lack of a coherent theory of sublimation remains one of the lacunae in psychoanalytic thought.

---

3 Note Rubinfine's (1961, pp. 84–85) summary: 'When such an image is formed, and represents a percept or memory trace thereof which has a conflicting affective charge (that is, painful and pleasurable, good and bad) and a strong drive cathexis, there is conflict as to whether to seek out and approach, or to avoid and withdraw . . . It is this kind of conflict which results via processes of displacement and condensation in the formation of a symbolic representation.' Notable exceptions include Segal (1957) and, apparently, Bernfeld (Bergmann, 1987).

4 For a sophisticated reading within the classical tradition, see Gross and Rubin (1973, p. 357): 'Sublimation is not a defense mechanism per se; it facilitates rather than opposes drive discharge. However, since it results in conflict solution by redirecting direct drive pressure via aim deflection, it can be said to have a defensive function.'

5 Hartmann (1964, p. 224) speaks of sublimation as a continuing life experience: 'If we agree with Freud's later proposition, we will tend to see sublimation not as a more or less occasional happening but rather a continuous process, which, of course, does not exclude temporary increases or decreases in sublimatory activities.'

Winnicott's (1971) understanding of cultural enterprises as out-
growths from the potential play space of childhood, making possible
in adulthood the sharing of necessary illusions, fills the lacuna that
Laplanche and Pontalis speak of. Winnicott's thesis is that only with
the experience of shared illusions, as exemplified in such activities as
art, philosophy, history, among others, can an individual feel real, as
well as related, and attain a sense of personal vitality. Within this
framework, symbol and sublimation are positively related, i.e., symbolism does not represent a failure of sublimation.[6]

Winnicott's (1958) approach to the symbolic process and sublimation arose out of his reflections on his work with patients who had not
yet achieved what he terms an integrated level of personalization. To
appreciate his perspective, a few comments on his technical style may
prove helpful. In such cases, Winnicott cautions analysts to provide a
therapeutic holding environment, rather than primarily an interpretive stance.

The holding environment is a rather sophisticated concept.
Winnicott meant it as a metaphor implying that patients have to feel
cared for before they can be careful, as well as ultimately carefree, with
themselves. Achievement of 'integration' and 'personalization' with the
presence of what Winnicott calls the 'True Self' involves the analytic
situation becoming analogous to the potential space between mother
and child or, in other words, a safe place of play. It is this safe place of
play that originally allows for the emergence of transitional objects and
transitional phenomena. The term 'transitional' refers to a specific type
of use of an object, or a repetitious behavior pattern, that serves as a
bridge between the experienced subjective self and the outside (maternal) objective world. Within this conceptual approach, the capacity to
form and use symbols becomes possible not primarily as a result of the
complexity of the individual's ego development, which makes repression and displacement possible, but rather of the experience and
developmental achievement of personal relating. (A significant developmental stage has been reached, Winnicott (1971) reminds us, when

---

6   Note Noy (1969, p. 176b): 'As the secondary process has to detach itself in the course of devel-
    opment from personal meanings and become more and more objective, the primary process
    has to improve its ability to deal with these personal meanings, i.e., become more and more
    subjective. So, each one has to develop in a different direction – but of course to the same
    degree'. Noy (1969, p. 157b) also writes: 'As the theory of regression, in the service of the ego,
    was created to integrate the view of artistic creativity as a superior ability within the psycho-
    analytic theory of the primitiveness of the primary process, it stands or falls with this last
    theory.'

the child is able both to relate to and to use the object and consequently integrate the *object mother* with the *environmental mother*.) Continuous personal connectedness, especially in the form of language, sustains the symbolic capacity in humans.

For Winnicott, inner phantasy constructs and outer reality are inextricably connected. Building on Winnicott's thoughts, I have suggested that mind is an experience *between* people rather than *in* people.[7] Note Winnicott's (1971, p. 96) observations about play:

> I realized, however, that *play is in fact neither a matter of inner psychic reality nor a matter of external reality* . . . I have claimed that when we witness an infant's employment of a transitional object, the first not-me possession, we are witnessing both the child's first use of a symbol and the first experience of play.

Such an approach grounds, in a developmental model, what we have always intuitively known about art, music, theater, for example, i.e., they function as a meeting place enabling people to relate to each other's subjectivity rather than operationally relating to each other's objectivity. Van Gogh's art gives us permission, as it were, to speak about and to know the irrational within us. Such cultural productions are communicative experiences, bridges between inner and outer. This can be true, for example, of some uses of religious myths; they can function as communal meaning-giving experiences that are complementary, not antagonistic, to any repressed sexual or aggressive meanings they may or may not contain.[8] As potential meaning-giving experiences, they reflect an interaction between an individual and society that is both normative and necessary for cultural life. Within this positive understanding of meaning-giving myths, we can certainly include psychoanalysis. Such experiences are, in effect, products of, as well as constitutive of, the play space where mind as a communicative phenomenon is manifest. That self and social communications can become more precise and fulfilling is one of the entertaining possibilities of human history. (Winnicott, 1971, speaks of psychoanalysis as a contemporary manifestation of play.)

We can understand sublimation, consequently, as closely related, if not identical, to the symbolic use of objects in this place of play, manifested by the capacity to play. Symbol, in this context, is that which

---

7 For a discussion of mind and its 'location', so to speak, see Chapters 2–4.
8 See, for example, the work of Eliade (1954, 1959, 1963, 1969) as well as Campbell (1979) for a sophisticated appreciation of the role of myth in human consciousness and community.

functions as a bridge, as we have said, between inner and outer realities.[9] Ideally, therefore, sublimation starts in the first year and progressively continues throughout an individual's life. It is the capacity to adaptively use symbols at different developmental levels, i.e., in a way that makes play, as Winnicott understands it, possible.[10] Note Winnicott (1965, p. 146) in this regard:

> The True Self has spontaneity, and this has been joined up with the world's events. The infant can now begin to enjoy the *illusion* of omnipotent creating and controlling, and then can gradually come to recognize the illusory element, the fact of playing and imagining. Here is the basis for the symbol which at first is *both* the infant's spontaneity or hallucination, *and also* the external object created and ultimately cathected.
>
> In between the infant and the object is some-thing, or some sensation. Insofar as this joins the infant to the object (viz. maternal part-object) so far is this the basis of symbol-formation. On the other hand, insofar as this something separates instead of joins, so is its function of leading on to symbol formation blocked.[11]

Winnicott here is more interested in describing the process out of which symbols come to be than in giving an academic, abstract definition. For the patient who has not yet achieved personal integration, i.e., the experience of feeling real and spontaneous, the primary task of the analytic process is to make (symbolic) play possible. A patient's progressive capacity to use language metaphorically is one example of this. The goal of analysis is, as we have always known, the capacity to experience sublimation.

---

9   Note, in particular, the work of Deri (1978).
10 In 1971, I wrote: 'in view of the growing understanding and integration into theory of the adaptive perspective which we have outlined and in conjunction with Noy's reading of the primary and secondary processes, there is evidence for a contemporary Freudian understanding of symbolic representation, for example, art, in other than regressive categories' (Gargiulo, 1971b, p. 160).
11 After completing this article I became aware of a vignette mentioned in Bergmann (1987) where he quotes from Jane Goodall (1971) a story relating her early interest in chimpanzees. The question, however, remains about the most informative model: did Goodall sublimate her transitional object (p. 153), as Bergmann suggests, following what I believe is the classical tradition, informed by ego psychology? Or did Goodall's age-appropriate and beneficial 'use' of her transitional chimp, reflecting her play space with her mother, prepare her for the creative use of her continuously growing adaptive functions? Bergmann also paraphrases Bernfeld's writing as follows: 'he recommended that sublimation be used neutrally for all instances where sexual wishes are diverted to serve the aims of the ego without regard to whether they serve important cultural purposes' (in Bergmann, 1987, p. 153). This is a position that I am obviously in agreement with, the significant difference being the source of sublimation, i.e., sexual wishes as diverted.

In *Playing and Reality* (1971), Winnicott notes, 'cultural experiences are in direct continuity with play, the play of those who have not yet heard of games' (p. 38). By contrast, 'failure of dependability or loss of object means to the child a loss of the play area, and loss (consequently) *of meaningful symbol*' (p. 38). Play, as noted above, means that in this potential space the child does not have to hold the self together but can let him- or herself go, as it were, in order to re-find him- or herself again at a new moment, achieving a new capacity to experience and express him- or herself as real and spontaneous rather than as simply compliant to external expectations. This is a place where *make-believe* is possible, where role-playing becomes fun without becoming engulfing or overwhelming: a place, to echo Winnicott's transitional object theme, where teddy bears accomplish great feats, and where no one asks who made the teddy bear. Winnicott (1971, pp. 96–97) writes:

> The object is a symbol of the union of the baby and the mother (or part of the mother). This symbol can be located. It is at the place in space and time where and when the mother is in transition from being (in the baby's mind) merged in with the infant and alternatively being experienced as an object to be perceived rather than conceived of.
>
> The use of an object symbolized the union of two now separate things, baby and mother, *at the point in time and space of the initiation of their state of separateness.*

Culture, as a particularly human possibility, can be seen as an outgrowth from these primal experiences. In this potential space 'between the subjective object and the object objectively perceived, between me-extensions and the not me' (Winnicott, 1971, p. 100), the child has intense experiences. The cultural life of any person has its roots in this potential space and, implicitly, in the adaptive or non-adaptive mothering environment; a place 'where separation . . . is not a separation but a form of union' (Winnicott, 1971, p. 98). A person's capacity to use and enjoy metaphor, as previously indicated, is directly related to achieving playful experiences rather than excessively concrete experiences.

Ricoeur (1970, p. 497) states, 'insofar as revealing and disguising coincide in it we might say that sublimation is the symbolic function itself'. What Ricoeur is suggesting here, in his phenomenological study of Freud's thought, is what Winnicott conceptualizes developmentally in his understanding of the potential transitional space between mother and child, i.e., in the shared moments of separation achieved, and yet union playfully (transitionally) regained, we have the playground that is the seedbed out of which symbolic experience grows and with it the experience of sublimation.[12] With Winnicott's understanding of *potential space*, we have a developmental as well as a theoretical understanding of symbol and of the ingredients of the maternal environment that make the symbolic process possible.

As I have indicated before, 'sublimation progressively occurs and is synonymous with achieving a capacity for adaptive symbolic behavior' (Gargiulo, 1976). In this regard, we may note that, when Segal (1957) speaks of 'symbols becoming available for sublimation' (p. 395), she does not join the two; furthermore, she speaks of the symbol in terms of reparation and the overcoming of loss through a displacement model approach:

> When this symbolic relation to faeces and other body products has been established, a projection can occur on to substances in the external world such as paint, plasticine, clay, etc., which can be used for sublimation.
>
> Segal (1957, p. 395a)[13]

Sublimation refers to the harmonious functioning of the subjective self with the created and creating environment so that *shared illusions* do not refer to private madness but have a communal participatory meaning. No one, for example, questions the astronomical or visual accuracy of Van Gogh's *Starry Night*, yet each person who responds to this masterpiece feels connected with the artist on some level and with his or her particular interpretation of reality. This is one example of what Winnicott means by play creating a shared world for human connectedness.

In summary, we can say that what is a particularly productive model for understanding cultural achievements is the facilitating maternal

---

12 Note Hacher (1972, p. 220): 'If man's symbolic equipment and its use is considered on a par with his instinctual endowment and his in-built ego apparatus, then sublimation signifies the successful (and at times socially valuable) employment of primary originary modes of expression based on the symbolic capacity and activity which as such needs no extraneous social and moral justification.' Although this is a position I am essentially in agreement with, Hacher is limited by his use of traditional metapsychology. That is, he states the very issue he should be explaining, namely, symbolic equipment.

13 Ogden (1985) builds on Segal's insights and combines them with Winnicott's in his discussion of the structural components of symbol formation: the symbol, the symbolized, and the thinker. He further develops symbol formation and the concept of projective identification but does not apply his conclusion about playing to the concept of sublimation.

holding environment. It is out of this experience of the potential space between mother and child, the play area between the *me* and the *not me*, that the capacity to interact creatively with one's personal and cultural milieu can arise. It is the emotional and psychical conditions of this play area that make sublimation possible. Winnicott's experience of humans as playful (*homo ludens*) enabled him to create a playground where culture and personal consciousness mirror each other. Other visions of humanity – tragic humans, guilty humans – offer other experiences of mind and humanity and consequently different conclusions.

The experience of sublimation, in its fullest expression, is the experience of living productively, living out the potential of the true self: the ability to experience a capacity for centeredness, an experience of being personally alive as well as competently effective. It is in the experience of playing in and with the world that one's potential for human fulfillment is most realized. Winnicott (1971, p. 103) highlights this when he writes:

> The potential space between baby and mother, between child and family, between individual and society or the world, depends on experiences which lead to trust. It can be looked upon as sacred to the individual in that it is here that the individual experiences creative living.

SECTION 4
CONCLUDING THOUGHTS

CHAPTER 12

A psychoanalytic/spiritual adventure

At a time when some physicists speculate about whether or not time exists, and when the journal *Scientific American* dedicates a lead article entitled 'Infinite earths in parallel universes really exist', technological man is beginning to understand that a positivistic, empirical world-view needs to be broadened, if we want to appreciate who and where we are.[1] In my focus on the need to be comfortable with mystery, with poetry, with unknowing, I have attempted to highlight the different dimensions that psychoanalysts must bring to clinical work, if they are going to know who and where they are. Throughout the text I have alluded to the works of Meister Eckhart to suggest a broader reading of what it means to be human.[2] None of this should stand in opposition to analysts understanding the genetic determinants of a person's present situation, nor does it exclude a sensible analysis of defenses or transference manifestations. What it suggests, however, is that, if analysts do the very things they are trained to do without appreciating a wider life context, i.e., what I have spoken of as a natural or everyday transcendence, they will miss something crucial in human experience.

Determinism, either psychological or cultural, has to be contextualized by an awareness of what quantum mechanics speaks of as *a mist of infinite possibilities*, and, as I hope I have made clear, I relate that to an awareness of an everyday transcendence. What that suggests to me, if we are going to know who we are, is a quiet openness to individual experience, a depth of appreciation that one must bring to the human enterprise, despite the repeated senseless cruelty we periodically visit

---

1 See Barbour (1999), as well as Tegmark (2003).
2 See Panikkar (1979) and Bobrow (1997) for a discussion of these traditions and their relationship to contemporary reflections in both theoretical physics as well as psychoanalysis.

on each other. A quiet openness to individual experience, or what can also be characterized as *a sensitivity to interiority*, is the ground place for any resolution of conflict and easing of psychological pain. It is the soil out of which grows the sense of dignity we owe ourselves. We should not only appreciate what Philip Rieff (1966) has so aptly called *twentieth-century psychological man*, but we can also look at our history through ancient eyes, so to speak, be they the eyes of the great prophets of the Hebrew scriptures, the insights of the Buddha, the teachings of Jesus, or the lessons of many spiritual guides who have walked among us. Whenever we change our metaphors, whenever we put on new lenses, we have the opportunity to see what we were not able to see before. Thus my repeated quotation from John Wheeler and others 'that the questions we ask determine the answers we get' (in Gliedman, 1984, p. 96).[3] With new lenses we can appreciate the Hebrew prophets' conviction that that which they called God is truly close by, the Buddha's teaching on enlightenment and compassion, Jesus' insistence on our radical equality and need to care for each other, as well as the mystics' focus on our profound ignorance of the *ground of being* that supports us.

Although I have spoken of psychoanalysis and spirituality as two different *histories of questioning*, they both address a vital emptiness that spiritual traditions have been more comfortable articulating than has psychoanalysis. Attentive to the possibility that, in speaking about the oneness of things or the non-existence of time, an individual might be suffering from a schizophrenic disorder (e.g., 'Mother and I are one'), psychoanalysis has ignored a possible different hearing of such themes. That some spiritual authors, on their side, have been equally inattentive to the pathological possibilities of the abuse of their teachings balances the record, so to speak. What both traditions have to be constantly vigilant about is falling into facts, into what Whitehead so aptly characterizes as misplaced concreteness, or, more prosaically, missing the forest for the trees. Facts should not distract the psychoanalyst, be they the facts of a patient's history, culture, defenses, or goals; taken in themselves, they are no guarantee that a patient, to quote Winnicott again, is alive.

That an individual, walking either a spiritual pilgrimage or a psychoanalytic journey, may be washed over by grief or rage, by unnamable anxiety or unbearable darkness, should not distract one

---

3 For a more detailed discussion see Wheeler et al. (1973).

from the goal of aliveness. The experience of personal creativity is ultimately the goal of both psychoanalytic and spiritual quests. It is better, in poetic imagery, to dance with God than to sleep with death. If we allow ourselves to ponder the possibility of a transcendent vital emptiness, understood in terms of *non-existence,* we will begin to sense the reality of mystery, i.e., what I have referred to as a pervasive inviting silence, an ever-receding horizon to our knowledge, the experience of mystery with which we live. It is out of this inviting silence, in the passing moments of life when one is able to experience it, that one finds the strength to be alive – an aliveness that is not simply a personal possession but a shared experience, an aliveness that has its roots in what we have spoken of as an everyday or natural transcendence.

I don't think it an exaggeration to state that the continuous noise we live with (cell/mobile phones, portable CD players, televisions, walkabout radios, etc.), contributes not just to efficacy but, all too frequently, to a dulling of awareness of interiority. When interiority is eclipsed, we extend the shadows we walk through, i.e., what I have spoken of as our 'ground space' is more difficult to experience when such distractions surround us. It is because we humans have a need to experience an everyday transcendence that we have such paths as psychoanalysis and spiritual journeys. Although the role of a therapist or analyst is not that of a teacher, an essential outcome of the therapeutic setting is for a patient to find his or her personal honesty and thereby create personal meaning. Such experiences are not just solitary accomplishments opening one up to one's forgotten history and/or unrecognized defenses; rather they make possible an experience of meeting the world, and others, on level ground.

Michelangelo's Sistine Chapel fresco of God creating man depicts them as finger close yet worlds apart. In reality, what touches us, what gives life to us, is the open-ended depth of the world and of ourselves as part of such an open-ended depth. Such openness does not entail either creedal beliefs or specific spiritual exercises. It does entail a quiet experience of mystery, an awareness of awe, an acceptance of the dignity we owe the world and ourselves.

A modern dialogue with Freud

Freud and philosophy

Ricoeur's 1970 text is both a provocative philosophical enterprise and a masterful reading of Freud, in which he analyses such questions as the meaning of psyche, the function of symbol and the reality of Eros. Although Ricoeur suggests some conclusions about these questions that must be critically examined, the work evidences a dignity of scholarship not readily seen today. As it is a text of extraordinary complexity and sensitivity, my analysis is inevitably somewhat cursory. The text is divided into three books, respectively, entitled: I, The Problematic: The Placing of Freud; II, Analytic: Reading of Freud; and III, Dialectic: A Philosophical Interpretation of Freud.

For Ricoeur, the problem that one must experience in order to place and evaluate the thought of Freud derives from the apparently opposing functions of interpretation, understood in its most generic sense: interpretation as a vehicle for recollection of meaning, i.e., revealer of the sublime or sacred, or interpretation as an exercise of suspicion in the sense of decipherer of the repressed. By way of introductory classification, Ricoeur places the religious concept of exegesis in the role of revealer of the sacred, whereas psychoanalysis becomes an exemplar of a reductionistic, secular, exegetical approach. The author begins with this level of understanding, although as the text develops it is subject to provocative and deeper readings. In this section Ricoeur outlines the specificity of symbol as container of double meaning, encompassing overt as well as covert meaning areas, which it is the specific aim of interpretation to decipher. With this basic understanding of symbol he begins the task of deciphering mind conceptualized within the Freudian model as force and meaning, i.e., as desire in search of interpretation. But, if interpretation ultimately reveals the sacred and/or if interpretation unmasks the hidden, how is one to know the path free from illusion? Aware of the delicacy of the task he has set for himself, Ricoeur quickly delimits the scope of consciousness, i.e., the possibility of a false consciousness that equates mind with a simplistic understanding of 'I think, therefore I am'. Such a cautionary move, however, brings him to his second book, Freud proper and psychoanalysis, the discipline of listening to mind.

Before going on to the second book, we might note that there is a certain initial polemical tone in Ricoeur's contrasting the functions of interpretation as revealing the sacred, and exercising suspicion in unmasking the hidden. Philip Rieff (1966) in *The Triumph of the Therapeutic* has also approached this problematic area through an analysis of what he calls the different theories of theory. Contrasting the religious individual and psychological individual, which designate for him historical/cultural consciousness, Rieff sees human expectation of the function of theory as necessarily formative of human findings. Thus, in an understanding of the role of theory that sees its generic function as progressively revealing reality up to a highest being, one is able to speak of transcendental truth, of unchanging reality, of God. In an alternative understanding of the role of theory in human conceptualizing, theory serves the role of helping individuals to organize their particular historical situation so that it functions better for them and thus meets their needs. The problem of the delineation of human knowledge, which Rieff responds to in terms of his two theories of theory, Ricoeur confronts with his developed study of symbolism. Yet, as will be indicated later, Ricoeur does not seem to be aware of Rieff's type of approach to this epistemological issue. Before developing his theory of symbolism, however, Ricoeur confronts Freud and his attempts to map consciousness, which becomes the subject matter of the second book.

A major criterion for psychoanalytic competence is whether the writer has integrated into his perspective such classic texts as Freud's 'Scientific Project' (Freud, 1896–1899), Chapter 7 of *The Interpretation of Dreams*, and his essays 'The Unconscious, the Ego, and the Id' and 'Beyond the Pleasure Principle'. Ricoeur not only studies these sources in detail but integrates them with a view of Freud's progressive development. Throughout the second book, he shows both sophistication and depth in his philosophical reading of Freud and psychoanalysis. The latter is especially noteworthy because Ricoeur confesses in the preface that his work might suffer from his not being an analyst. Nevertheless, there are few American analysts or therapists writing today who take such care to master Freud before entering into a dialogue with him. Ricoeur employs a phenomenological methodology that makes this section on Freud, condensed as it is, unfold with a graceful internal consistency.

From Freud's earliest models of the psyche, using mechanical analogs, to his ripened thought on the battle between Eros and Thanatos, he set himself the task of listening to the mind. His first studies suggest a solipsistic model, but, as is clear to anyone who reads beneath the surface, Freud understands instinct or, to use Ricoeur's insightful term, desire, as directed toward another person. Indeed, for Ricoeur, primal repression flows from the very structure of desire insofar as desire is from the very beginning confronted by another desire. Thus, in the topographical model of the mind (conscious, preconscious, and unconscious), not only does Freud establish system models with which to designate the many tributaries inherent in mind, but he also traces instinct understood as desire in its search for meaning. Ultimately, it is because desire has semantics, as Ricoeur repeatedly shows, that Freud speaks about the *instinctual representatives* as being the object of his science. The ever-present biological force is a force that, in humans, becomes desire, and thus there is the possibility of mind.

In studying the different vicissitudes of the instinctual representatives, be they manifested in ideas or affects, Freud posits the unconscious, preconscious, and conscious as tools for an archeology of the mind. In 1923, when he presents his structural model of ego, id, and superego, it is because desires may be mapped not only in regard to place, as it were, but also in respect to an individual's personal history and his or her experiences with love and authority. Thus the drama of roles must be explicitly incorporated into one's perspective if one wishes to listen to mind more fully – and the roles are the personal (ego), the impersonal (id), and the suprapersonal (superego).

In the id, there is the constant presence of desires, for the ego the task of a dialogue with personal time, and in the superego the burden of cultural history. In the unfolding of this drama of roles there is the gradual pain of recognition as id learns, so to speak, that it is not ego. And by not fleeing from the rendezvous with love and authority the ego progressively develops not only spontaneity of desire (pleasure principle) but also a capacity to hold desires within, while mastering the script of the historical moment (reality principle). Freud has, however, many thoughts on reality, as Ricoeur makes clear. Before discussing these, we must turn to the role of psychoanalytic interpretation understood within the drama of the psyche just mentioned.

Interpretation is a meaning-giving process of deciphering the hidden in the present. Interpretation takes place in time and, because the psyche plays its drama for an audience, interpretation is always personalized. Thus arises the psychoanalytic understanding of transference and the valid perspective on interpretation, which Ricoeur presents: that psychoanalytic experience is simply not an observable science as so many academic psychologists endeavor to see it. It cannot be verified, as in physical and experimental sciences, with a measurable degree of reliability, not because it is a defective science but because its subject matter is personalized history as presented by one consciousness to another. The other is a second consciousness trained to listen to the drama with minimal intrusiveness and to communicate what he or she sees, what he or she experiences, to the player. For one might view neurosis as a player reciting lines endlessly in search of their meaning. Neurosis and the more pathological conflicts are, accordingly, symbolic distortions of childhood desires and demands that cannot leave the scene until they have found a meaning. As the analyst selects one avenue to search for personal meaning, Ricoeur sees psychoanalysis as more akin to history and thus not readily reproducible in the psychologist's laboratory. Furthermore, because interpretation deciphers the dynamic unconscious – tracing the historical fluctuations of desire – it is not reducible to phenomenology either.

After studying the complexity of the psychic systems and aware of the ever-present narcissism of which the mind is a child, Ricoeur ventures into an understanding of truth and its possible delimitation. This brings us to the third book, Ricoeur's philosophical reflections on symbol and the meaning of reality vis-à-vis Eros, *Ananke* (necessity), and Thanatos.

Returning to the tension indicated in the first book, between the respective functions of interpretation as revealer of the sacred and *unmasker* of the hidden, Ricoeur presents a detailed study of the complex psychoanalytic concept of sublimation and its relation to symbol. Substantially differing from the other vicissitudes that desires undergo, sublimation not only changes, in technical terms, the aim of a particular drive but in addition to its successful achievement signals a new organization of consciousness, one productive of new meaning. Ricoeur presents Freud's thought on art as the clearest example of this, and he uses these thoughts to unite the concepts of symbolization and sublimation. Within such a context, symbols can be seen as having both an archeology and a teleology, i.e., they contain both regressive hidden dimensions and progressive and new historical meaning. Ricoeur's thesis is that authentic symbols must be both a locus of the repressed – the hidden – of the childhood conflicts that stamp the historical development of mind, and a harbinger of the highest historical insights of human consciousness – the *sublime or the sacred*, to use the author's words. This approach to symbol, it seems to me, is comparable to the work Erikson has done on the concept of identity in both its regressive dimensions and its progressive or epigenetic development. Identity, for Erikson, is like a two-edged sword cutting into the hidden past and, out of that very past, forging a new future.

In this connection it is important to realize that Freud's concentration on the regressive, the unmasking, was not because he denied the possibility of the progressive but because he considered sublimation, which is not a repressive process, as non-neurotic. In Freud's writing on psychic determinism, he notes that analysis can decipher the past but cannot therefore predict a future. Ricoeur seems aware of this because he notes that it is one of the rarely articulated premises on which psychoanalytic therapy relies. Humans are capable of understanding themselves, of reinterpreting their fantasies and of finding their true historical self. Having done that, the burden of the past is significantly lighter and they will be better able to love and to work. Having said this, we must note that necessity, or *Ananke* as Ricoeur refers to it, is certainly not mere adaptation or resignation to reality, although it is that. Rather, by experiencing this at a deeper level, the individual develops a recognition and acceptance of the unchangeableness of the history he or she has lived.

In Eriksonian terms, this becomes recognition of the inevitability of the human lifecycle and a need to achieve the self-understanding that can give new *liberating meaning* to the life experiences one has had. These are not closure concepts but simply limit concepts, and through these Erikson masterfully brings to the fore authentic but latent thoughts of Freud. It is the achievement of the truth of one's history that is the most creative reading of the psychoanalytic concept of the reality principle. The reality principle does not refer merely to the recognition of external facts but even more to the truth of internal history. Free from repeating the past, libido – the child of Eros – is able to love with minimal oppression from the superego. Finally, throughout most of the text, Ricoeur is aware that in the battle of the giants Freud opts, in his cautious and analytic way, for Eros.

In the closing sections of the work, Ricoeur moves to a more critical position in reference to Freud. In his analysis of different types of symbols, he highlights the *prospective symbol*, those symbols that point to the horizon stretching before man's spiritual or consciousness quest. (This is in contradistinction to those symbols that reflect the opposite horizon, as it were, separating man from his childhood.) These final chapters consist of a highly condensed study that involves primarily Hegelian models; their underlying assumption is that a theory of mind may enable one to reach ultimate and/or sacred reality. In this sense, Ricoeur is in the primary tradition of western philosophy and theology, and his flight to the inexplicableness of the symbolism of evil as a reminder of the supposed gaps in human knowledge is at least consistent. The issues involved in this discussion are too complex to resolve here, for ultimately Ricoeur is speaking about the experience of value in human consciousness. Yet the objectivity of value can be respected, it seems to me, without recourse to a particular reading of the symbolism of evil understood as indicating man's created and/or redeemable state. For to say that humans are incomplete is to comment on our historicity, to notice defects is to appreciate evolution, and to speak of evil is to be aware that power, in its many forms, may go astray.

As Ricoeur apparently must go beyond the value of such prospective symbols that are reflected in art, together with their capacity to raise human consciousness, he postulates, in his discussion of the unfolding horizons, the presence of the sacred, the *wholly other*. And as noted above he seems surprisingly unaware of the epistemological model he is using, which ultimately allows him to make such postulates.

Thus the final pages of the text become more understandable but not any less disappointing in a work of such excellence. For we must finally note that, contrary to what one might expect, Ricoeur speaks of Freud's understanding of the reality principle predominately in terms of resignation, apparently overruling his own readings of that very concept which go beyond such a narrow interpretation. Consequently he sets up a dichotomy between *Ananke* and Eros that is a false one, for Freud and psychoanalysis are no philistine disciples of *Ananke*, understood as mere resignation. Rather, the analytic discipline, at its best, can free a man to find love, but it stops short, and consciously so, of naming that love or of committing the patient to a commitment. But it does this in order that individuals can, with some measure of autonomy, name themselves.

Who is the dreamer who dreams the dream?

A study of psychic presences

In an engrossing poem entitled 'I am not even dust', Jorges Luis Borges ends with the prayer that his god, his dreamer, 'keep on dreaming' him (Borges, 1999, p. 401). Most North American analysts would dismiss this last line, in particular, as religious mysticism, a left-over from a pre-differentiated developmental stage, something to be resolved and not celebrated. John Gedo (1999), in *The Evolution of Psychoanalysis,* goes so far as to state that recent neurological findings suggest that dreams have no meaning at all, implying that to attribute meaning to them is a *mentalist presupposition* unworthy of a scientific, biologically grounded, psychoanalysis (p. 204). While making a didactically clear and at times persuasive argument, Gedo's position, as I read him, ignores our metaphorical modes of thinking as well as our culturally dependent awareness of a beyond in our midst, a beyond that has been articulated in terms of transcendence – either the absolute transcendence, which western religious traditions have highlighted, or the relative everyday experience of transcendence, which Grotstein studies in his attempt to locate the dreamer who dreams the dream.

In a tour de force entailing a reading of Freud, Jung, Lacan, Klein, Winnicott, Heidegger, Matte-Blanco, and Bion, among others, Grotstein (2000) posits the basic function of the dream as a communication between what he categorized as *the ineffable subject of the unconscious* (the dreamer who dreams the dream) and *the dreamer who understands the dream.* He sets himself the task of decoding, for lack of a better word, the psychic presences that reflect and/or deflect the ineffable subject of the unconscious. Grotstein (2000, p. xxiv) writes:

. . . the task of psychoanalysis is not the attainment of insight but, rather, the use of insight to attain transcendence over oneself, over one's masks and disguises, to rebecome one's supraordinate subject. This task involves a transcendent reunion with one's ineffable subject in a moment of aletheia (unconcealment).

Grotstein grapples with the psyche's mystery and comprehensibility; his work should be read, I believe, as more in the tradition of theoretical physics than Gedo's biological neurology. Comprehensibility and mystery are not necessarily antagonistic concepts – note Einstein's reflection 'the eternal mystery of the world is its comprehensibility' (in Gregory, 1988, p.189).

The text is dense with awareness, not afraid to approach mysterious or mythological themes from a psychoanalytic perspective, Grotstein has given us a text more akin to an evocative poem – a work that has to be read quietly and, for some sections, repeatedly. As Thomas Ogden writes in his preface, which offers an extremely helpful synthesizing overview, one cannot summarize a poem without reproducing it. One might, therefore, characterize this work as a text poem.

Following Melanie Klein as his most useful model, with acknowledged updating from Ogden, Grotstein builds his case by fleshing out the psychoanalytic ramifications of his various theses. In revisiting his notion of autochthony – *the fantasy of self-creation* – Grotstein offers an insightful and appealing reinterpretation of the Adam and Eve myth. Further expanding his perspective, he uses this concept to gain a better appreciation of trauma. Following Winnicott's thoughts on trauma as an intrusion into the psyche before a person is allowed to personally create the found world, Grotstein explains, in some detail, how persecutors have to be turned into enemies. Grotstein frees Kleinian thought from the confines of its informing specific and concretized developmental states; he does this by helping us appreciate the ageless child that is our companion throughout life.

Although Grotstein gives a flexible and creative reading of Klein, he occasionally suggests a level of verification not possible for psychoanalytic concepts. He writes, for example, of 'Klein's discovery of projective identification' (Grotstein, 2000, p. xxii). He is certainly not alone in this mode of speaking, e.g., analysts frequently speak of Freud's *discovery* of the unconscious or his *discovery* of the meaning of dreams, thereby inadvertently eclipsing an appreciation of the metaphorical nature of psychoanalytic concepts.

In this context I have elsewhere noted:

> Ultimately, then, it makes no sense to believe in anything if that means for-getting the metaphorical nature of knowledge. Sir Peter Medawar (1982), the English research biologist and philosopher, is not alone when he reminds us that even in the empirical sciences 'a hypothesis is an imaginative precon-ception of what might be true.' . . . Understanding the metaphorical basis of knowledge frees us of the Herculean burden of finding *the* truth. We can, instead, settle for a truth, or should I say several truths.
>
> Gargiulo (1998a, pp. 418–419)[1]

It is in light of these obvious considerations that I read such authors as Bion, Klein, or Winnicott, and their metaphorical encounter with the psyche's elusive complexity, and can subsequently read Grotstein's creative interpretations of them, among the many authors he studies.

By studying Grotstein's intelligent, clear, and informative reading of Bion, the reader is invited to reflect on the *beingness* that flows through us, an experience of which is the opposite of what Fingarette (1963) calls the anxious ego. Grotstein (2000, p. 282) speaks to this issue when he proffers his:

> . . . own idea of a 'transcendent position' to account for the state of seren-ity that accompanies one who finally, after traversing the nightmares of the paranoid-schizoid position and the black holes and mournful inner cathe-drals of the depressive position, is able to become reconciled to the expe-rience of pure, unadulterated Being and Happening.

In his psychoanalytic demythologizing of religious themes, Grotstein exemplifies a mode of thinking that echoes William James (1993) in *The Varieties of Experience*. The everyday transcendence of the indescribable or *ineffable* subject of the unconscious locates, in Grotstein's reading, the significance of the *God experience* and the *Christ experience*, among other myth themes. Such observations issue from a mode of thinking where the unknowable real, the transcendent 'O' that we are driven to find, are postulated as fundamental points of reference. Grotstein is not alone in this line of inquiry. His psychoan-alytic integration of these themes, however, places him in the forefront of analytic writers. Robert M. Torrance, a contemporary academic writer addressing transcendence in myth, religion, and science, writes:

---

1 Martin Heidegger notes 'that language is the House of being . . . the language we use tells the kind of world we can expect to find' (in Gregory, 1988, p. 199). This text is particularly help-ful for anyone wishing to understand how theoretical physics views theory and language.

... objective truth of religious experience thus lies not in a changeless entity outside or beyond the human but in the continuity or interrelation
between the individual and a kindred other – call it futurity, potentiality, or
spirit – through which the individual self is expanded.

Torrance (1994, pp. 284–285).

This is precisely Grotstein's goal: the expansion of the self and thereby an expansion of the other.

As is clear from the foregoing, this is not a text that can be summarized or easily characterized. This is a work of kaleidoscopic
complexity, as complex as the art of understanding ourselves.
Although psychoanalysts assume individuated subjectivity as the
locus of meaning and therefore of mind, there are other traditions
that have grappled with similar issues from different and illuminating
perspectives. On the contemporary scene, there is the work of Marcia
Cavell (1988) and, within a different intellectual milieu, the reflections of medieval philosophers. Although Cavell locates meaning as
coming from the community, Thomas Aquinas (1975, pp. 215–227)
and the Arabian philosopher Averroes argue as to whether there is
one source of meaning, one mind, so to speak, that informs the myr-
iad of human beings, or, as seems obvious, many minds (see Gilson,
1955, pp. 216–220; Copleston, 1993). This is not an idle observation,
as it might first appear. One mind locates the subject of meaning as
transcendent to the individual without being antagonistic to the individual. Zen Buddhism, which is not dissimilar to Averroes' teachings,
speaks of the illusion of the *I* or *ego* or achieving the experience of *no
mind*, all of which, paradoxically, grounds one in a deeper reality
(Gargiulo, 1997).

Struggling through the night, as it were, with the angels of preter-
natural psychic presences, Grotstein returns, repeatedly, to his theme
of the ineffable subject of the unconscious, wherein he locates meaning as both within and transcendent to the individual. I was reminded
of the difference between Groddeck's notions of the unconscious as
reflected in his *The Book of the It* (1976) and Freud's more neutralized
concept as reflected in his essay on *The Unconscious* (1915). Grotstein
is in the tradition of those who experience the unconscious as alive
and brimming over with creativity, not necessarily a seething cauldron
of the repressed and the instincts. One ramification that follows from
Freud's model is the somewhat exclusive focus of many analysts on
symptoms and defense, transference, and its resolution. Without an

expanded notion of the unconscious, however, and recognition of the unknowable real, and/or the 'O' of Bion, psychoanalysis can become an exercise in repetitive procedures, forgetting thereby that 'theory as practice is a living bridge between patient and analyst, which the analyst and patient construct, repetitively' (Gargiulo, 1989, p. 158).

As I mentioned earlier, this text does not lend itself to any overriding summary; it is too rich and complex for that. Feeling some constraint, nevertheless, to summarize, I would say that Grotstein's leitmotif is his explication of the *ineffable subject of the unconscious*, whereby two additional subjectivities, two more forgotten companions, have been brought to the analytic table. The Muse of the poet or the artist, the creative intuitions of everyday life, the experience of mystery and awe have been reintroduced for both patient and analyst in their search for self-understanding and their encounter with the real.

Borges seems relevant again. In his poem 'Borges and I', he notes, laconically, 'if, in fact, I am a self' (Borges, 1999, p. 93).[2] In this line, Borges reflects, I believe, his sense of a deeper self, an unconscious self that defines the conscious self – a conscious self that, in its ignorance, sees only itself, reflected in a mirror. Grotstein's *Who Is the Dreamer Who Dreams the Dream?* (2000) not only shows us why we must ponder such questions but also sets before us a path we can follow in our reflections.

---

2 For an interesting discussion of this theme, see Ogden (2000).

References

Aquinas, T. (1975). Summa Contra Gentiles, Vol. 2. London: Notre Dame Press.

Balint, M. (1965). Primary Love and Psychoanalytic Technique. New York: Liveright Publishing Corp.

Balint, M. (1979). The Basic Fault. New York: Brunner/Mazel, originally published 1968.

Barbour, J. (1999). The End of Time. Oxford: Oxford University Press.

Beller, M. (1999). Quantum Dialogue. Chicago: University of Chicago Press.

Bergmann, M.S. (1987) The Anatomy of Loving. New York: Columbia University Press.

Bobrow, J. (1997). Coming to life: The creative intercourse of psychoanalysis and Zen Buddhism. In: Spezzano, C. and Gargiulo, G. (eds), Soul on the Couch. Hillsdale, NJ: The Analytic Press.

Borges, J.L. (1999). Selected Poems (A. Coleman, ed.). New York: Penguin Books.

Bouveresse, J. (1995). Wittgenstein Reads Freud. Princeton: Princeton University Press.

Breuer, J. and Freud, S. (1893–1895). Studies on Hysteria (Standard edn, Vol. XI). London: Hogarth Press.

Brown, N.O. (1959). Life Against Death. New York: Vintage Books.

Brown, N.O. (1966). Love's Body. New York: Random House.

Calvino, I. (1974). Invisible Cities. New York: Harcourt Brace Janovich.

Campbell, J. (1979). The Hero with a Thousand Faces. Princeton: Princeton University Press.

Campbell, J. (1986). The Inner Reaches of Outer Space. New York: Harper & Row.

Capra, F. (1982). The Turning Point. New York: Bantam Books.

Cavell, M. (1988). Solipsism and community. Psychoanalysis and Contemporary Thought, 11(4).

Cavell, M. (1993). The Psychoanalytic Mind. Cambridge: Harvard University Press.

Chang, K. (2000). Here, there, and everywhere: a quantum state of mind. New York Times, July 11. Available at http://query.nytimes.com/gst/abstract.html?res=F10712F6395C0C728DDDAE0894D8404482.

Colledge, E. and McGinn, B. (1981). Meister Eckhart. New York: Paulist Press.

Copleston, F. (1993). A History of Philosophy, Vol. 2. New York: Doubleday.

Corrington, R.S. (1994). Ecstatic Naturalism. Indianapolis, IN: Indiana University Press.

Corrington, R.S. (1997). Nature's Religion. Oxford: Rowman & Littlefield.

Damasio, A. (2003). Looking for Spinoza. New York: Harcourt Books.

Deri, S. (1978). Transitional phenomena: Vicissitudes of symbolization and creativity. In: Grolnick, S. and Barkin, L. (eds), Between Reality and Fantasy. New York: Jason Aronson Press.

Einstein, A. (1954). Physics and reality. In: Ideas and Opinions. New York: Crown.

Eliade, M. (1954). Cosmos and History: The myth of the eternal return. New York: Harper & Row.

Eliade, M. (1959). The Sacred and the Profane. New York: Harper & Row.

Eliade, M. (1963). Myth and Reality. New York: Harper & Row.

Eliade, M. (1969). Images and Symbols. New York: Sheed & Ward.

Eliot, T.S. (1943). Four Quartets. New York: Harcourt Brace & Company.

Ellenberger, H.F. (1970). The Discovery of the Unconscious. New York: Basic Books.

Erikson, E. (1963). Childhood and Society. New York: W.W. Norton.

Erikson, E. (1964). Insight and Responsibility. New York: W.W. Norton.

Erikson, E. (1966). Ontogeny of ritualization. In: Loewenstein, R., Newman, L., Schur, M. and Solint, A. (eds), Psychoanalysis: A general psychology. New York: International Universities Press.

Fairbairn, R.D. (1954). An Object-Relations Theory of the Personality. New York: Basic Books.

Fenichel, O. (1945). The Psychoanalytic Theory of Neurosis. New York: W.W. Norton.

Ferenczi, S. (1988). The Clinical Diary of Sandor Ferenczi (J. Dupont, trans.). Cambridge, MA: Harvard University Press.

Fingarette, H. (1963). The Self in Transformation. New York: Harper & Row.

Freud, S. (1893–1895). Studies On Hysteria (Standard edn, Vol. II). London: Hogarth Press, 1955.

Freud, S. (1896–1899). Project for a Scientific Psychology (Standard edn, Vol. I). London: Hogarth Press, 1966.

Freud, S. (1901–1905). A Case of Hysteria (Standard edn, Vol. VII). London: Hogarth Press, 1953.

Freud, S. (1905). Three Essays on the Theory of Sexuality. (Standard edn, Vol. VI). London: Hogarth Press, 1953.

Freud, S. (1910). Five Lectures on Psychoanalysis (Standard edn, Vol. XI). London: Hogarth Press, 1957.

Freud, S. (1913). On Beginning Treatment: Further recommendations on the technique of psychoanalysis (Standard edn, Vol XII). London: Hogarth Press, 1958.

Freud, S. (1914). On Narcissism (Standard edn, Vol. XIV). London: Hogarth Press, 1957.

Freud, S. (1915). The Unconscious (Standard edn, Vol. XIV). London: Hogarth Press, 1957.

Freud, S. (1923). The Ego and the Id (Standard edn, Vol. XIX). London: Hogarth Press, 1961.

Freud, S. (1926). The Question of Lay Analysis (Standard edn, Vol. XX). London: Hogarth Press, 1959.

Freud, S. (1927). The Future of an Illusion (Standard edn, Vol. XXI). London: Hogarth Press, 1961.

Freud, S. (1930). Civilization and Its Discontents (Standard edn, Vol. XXI). London: Hogarth Press, 1961.

Freud, S. (1974). The Freud/Jung Letters (W. McGuire, ed.). Princeton: Princeton University Press.

Fromm, E., Suzuki, D.T. and DeMartino, R. (1960). Zen Buddhism and Psychoanalysis. New York: Harper & Row.

Gargiulo, G.J. (1971a). A modern dialogue with Freud. The Psychoanalytic Review, 58(2).

Gargiulo, G.J. (1971b). Theoretical models and the psychoanalytic understanding of symbols. Cross Currents (Spring), 155–163.

Gargiulo, G.J. (1979). The place of play. Newsletter of the Council of Psychoanalytic Psychotherapists, 1–6.

Gargiulo, G.J. (1984). Anna O.: An English object relations approach. In: Rosenbaum, M. and Melvin, M. (eds), Anna O.: Fourteen contemporary reinterpretations. New York: The Free Press.

Gargiulo, G.J. (1989). Authority, the self, and psychoanalytic experience. The Psychoanalytic Review, 76(2), 155–166.

Gargiulo, G.J. (1991). Reflections, musings, and interventions: A personal communication on psychoanalytic work. In: Thorne, E. and Schaye, S. (eds), Psychoanalysis Today. Springfield, IL: Charles Thomas Publishers.

Gargiulo, G.J. (1992). Sublimation: Winnicottian reflections. The Psychoanalytic Review, 79(3).

Gargiulo, G.J. (1997). Inner mind/outer mind and the quest for the 'I.' In: Spezzano, C. and Gargiulo, G. (eds), Soul on the Couch. Hillsdale, NJ: The Analytic Press.

Gargiulo, G.J. (1998a). Meaning and metaphor in psychoanalytic education. The Psychoanalytic Review, 85, 413–422.

Gargiulo, G.J. (1998b). Winnicott's psychoanalytic playground. In: Marcus, P. and Rosenberg, A. (eds), Psychoanalytic Versions of the Human Condition. New York: New York University Press.

Gargiulo, G.J. (1998c). Remembering a Quiet Place. In: Reppen, J. (ed.), Why I Became a Psychotherapist. London: Jason Aronson.

Gargiulo, G.J. (1999). Language, love, and healing: A psychoanalyst's perspective. Journal of Religion and Health, 38, 341–345.

Gargiulo, G.J. (2001). Who is the dreamer who dreams the dream? A review essay. The Psychoanalytic Review, 88, 483–488.

Gargiulo, G.J. (2002). Recollection, empathy, and reverie. In: Breggin, P.R., Breggin, G., Bemak, F. (eds), Dimensions of Empathic Therapy. New York: Springer Publications, Inc.

Gargiulo, G.J. (2004). Aloneness in psychoanalysis and spirituality. International Journal of Applied Psychoanalytic Studies, 1(1), 36–46.

Gedo, J. (1999). The Evolution of Psychoanalysis. New York: Other Press.

Gerhardi, W. (1981). God's Fifth Column. New York: Simon & Schuster.

Gilson, F. (1955). History of Christian Philosophy in the Middle Ages. New York: Random House.

Gliedman, J. (1984). Turning Einstein upside down. Science Digest (October).

Glover, E. (1963). Freud or Jung? New York: Meridian Books.

Goodall, J. (1971). In the Shadow of Man. Boston, MA: Houghton Mifflin Company.

Green, A. (1975). The analyst, symbolization, and absence in the analytic setting. International Journal of Psychoanalysis, 56, 1–22.

Greene, B. (2000). The Elegant Universe. New York: Vintage Books.

Gregory, B. (1988). Inventing Reality. New York: John Wiley & Sons.

Groddeck, G. (1976). The Book of It. New York: Vintage Books.

Gross, G. and Rubin, I. (1973). Sublimation. In: The Psychoanalytic Study of The Child, Vol. 27. New York: Quadrangle Books.

Grotstein, J.D. (1998). W.R.D. Fairbairn and his growing significance for psychoanalysis and psychotherapy. In: Marcus, P. and Rosenberg, A. (eds), Psychoanalytic Versions of the Human Condition. New York: New York University Press.

Grotstein, J.D. (2000). Who Is the Dreamer Who Dreams the Dream? Hillsdale, NJ: The Analytic Press.

Guntrip, H. (1973). Psychoanalytic Theory, Therapy, and the Self. New York: International Universities Press.

Hacher, F. (1972). Sublimation. International Journal of Psychoanalysis, 53, 219–223.

Harrison, E.R. (1981). Cosmology: The science of the universe. New York: Cambridge University Press.

Hartmann, H. (1964). Essays on Ego Psychology. New York: International Universities Press.

Hawking, S.W. (1988). A Brief History of Time. New York: Bantam Books.

Heidegger, M. (1977). Martin Heidegger: Basic writings (D. Krell, trans.). New York: Harper & Row.

Heidegger, M. (1996). Being and Time (J. Stambaugh, trans.). Albany, NY: State University of New York Press.

Heisenberg, W. (1999). Physics and Philosophy. Amherst: Prometheus Books.

Jacoby, R. (1983). The Repression of Psychoanalysis. New York: Basic Books.

Jacques, F. (1991). Difference and Subjectivity (A. Rothwell, trans.). New Haven, CT: Yale University Press.

James, W. (1993). The Varieties of Religious Experience. New York: Random House.

Johnson, A.H. (1963). Whitehead's Theory of Reality. New York: Dover Publications.

Jones, E. (1948). Collected Papers, 5th edn. London: Baillière Tindall.

Jones, E. (1953, 1955, 1957). The Life and Works of Sigmund Freud. New York: Basic Books.

Kerr, J. (1994). A Most Dangerous Method. New York: Vintage Books.

Khan, M.M. (1974). The Privacy of the Self. New York: International Universities Press.

Khan, M.M. (1975). Introduction to Winnicott's Collected Papers, Through Paediatrics to Psychoanalysis. London: Hogarth Press.

Kistler, W. (1995). Face of myself. In: Poems of the Known World. New York: Arcade Publishing.

Lacan, J. (1977). Ecrits. New York: W.W. Norton.

Laplanche, J. and Pontalis, J.B. (1973). The Language of Psycho-Analysis (D.N. Smith, trans.). New York: W.W. Norton.

Lear, J. (1990). Love and Its Place in Nature. New York: Farrar, Straus & Giroux.

Little, M. (1990). Psychotic Anxieties and Containment. Northvale, NJ: Jason Aronson Press.

Marcuse, H. (1955). Eros and Civilization. New York: Bantam Books.

McGinn, B. (2001). The Mystical Thought of Meister Eckhart. New York: Crossroad Publishing.

Medawar, P. (1982). Pluto's Republic. New York: Oxford University Press.

Merton, T. (1968). Zen and the Birds of Appetite. New York: New Directions.

Noy, P. (1969). A revision of the psychoanalytic theory of the primary process. International Journal of Psychoanalysis, 50, 155–177.

Ogden, T. (1985). On potential space. International Journal of Psychoanalysis, 66, 391–397.

Ogden, T. (2000). Borges and the Art of Mourning. Psychoanalytic Dialogues, No. 10.

Panikkar, R. (1979). Myth, Faith, and Hermeneutics. New York: Paulist Press.

Phillips, A. (1988). Winnicott. Cambridge, MA: Harvard University Press.

Pollock, G.H. (1968). The possible significance of childhood object loss in the Joseph Breuer–Bertha Pappenheim (Anna O.) Sigmund Freud's Relationship. Journal of the American Psychoanalytic Association, 16(4).

Przywara, E. (1958). An Augustine Synthesis. New York: Harper Torchbooks.

Reik, T. (1948). Listening with the Third Ear. New York: Grove Press.

Ricoeur, P. (1970). Freud and Philosophy. New Haven, CT: Yale University Press.

Ricoeur, P. (1981). Hermeneutics and the Human Sciences. Cambridge: Cambridge University Press.

Rieff, P. (1966). The Triumph of the Therapeutic. New York: Harper & Row.

Rodman, R. (1990). Insistence on being himself. In: Giovacchini, P. (ed.), Tactics and Techniques in Psychoanalytic Therapy, Vol. III. Northvale, NJ: Jason Aronson Press.

Romanyshyn, R. (1983). Psychological Life. Austin, TX: University of Texas Press.

Roustang, F. (1982). Dire Mastery. Baltimore, MD: Johns Hopkins University Press.

Roustang, F. (1983). Psychoanalysis Never Lets Go. Baltimore, MD: Johns Hopkins University Press.

Rubinfine, D.L. (1961). Perception, reality testing, and symbolism. In: The Psychoanalytic Study of the Child, Vol. 16. New York: International Universities Press.

Sandler, J. and Joffee, W.G. (1987). Sublimation. In: Sander, J. (ed.), From Safety to Superego. New York: The Guilford Press.

Sartre, J-P. (1937). The Transcendence of the Ego. New York: Farrar, Straus & Giroux.

Segal, H. (1957). Notes on symbol formation. International Journal of Psychoanalysis, 38, 391–397.

Tagore, R. (1949/1977). Collected Poems and Plays. New York: Macmillan.

Tegmark, M. (2003). Parallel universes. Scientific American, 288(5), 41–51.

Thomas, L. (1974). The Lives of a Cell. New York: Bantam Books.

Thomas, L. (1984). Late Night Thoughts on Listening to Mahler's Ninth Symphony. Toronto: Bantam Books.

Torrance, R.M. (1994). The Spiritual Quest: Transcendence in myth, religion, and science. Berkeley, CA: University of California Press.

Vergote, A. (1983). From Freud's 'other scene' to Lacan's 'other'. In: Smith, J. and Kerrigan, W. (eds), Interpreting Lacan. New Haven, CT: Yale University Press.

Wallace, A.B. (1996). Choosing Reality. New York: Snow Lion Publications.

Wheeler, J., Misner, C. and Thorne, K. (1973). Gravitation. San Francisco, CA: W.H. Freeman.

Whitehead, A.N. (1957). Process and Reality. New York: Harper & Row.

Whitehead, A.N. (1960). Religion in the Making. New York: Macmillan, originally published 1929.

Winnicott, C. (1989). D.W.W.: A Reflection. In: Winnicott, C., Shepherd, R. and Davis, M. (eds), Psycho-Analytic Explorations. Cambridge, MA: Harvard University Press.

Winnicott, D.W. (1957). The Child and the Family. London: Tavistock.

Winnicott, D.W. (1958). Collected Papers. London: Tavistock.

Winnicott, D.W. (1965). The Maturational Processes and the Facilitating Environment. New York: International Universities Press.

Winnicott, D.W. (1971). Playing and Reality. New York: Basic Books.

Winnicott, D.W. (1988). Human Nature. New York: Schocken Books.

Winnicott, D.W. (1989). Review of Memories, Dreams, Reflections. In: Winnicott, C., Shepherd, R. and Davis, M. (eds), Psycho-Analytic Explorations. Cambridge, MA: Harvard University Press.

Zukav, G. (1979). The Dancing Wu Li Masters. New York: William Morrow.

Index

Wiley The manufacturer's authorized representative according to the EU
General Product Safety Regulation is Wiley-VCH GmbH, Boschstr. 12,
69469 Weinheim, Germany, e-mail: Product_Safety@wiley.com.

Printed and bound by CPI Group (UK) Ltd, Croydon, CR0 4YY
17/12/2025
02021031-0002